# Our Conclusion

Thalassemia is not a genetic disorder; it is a man-made disease as a result of drugs, vaccination, misdiagnosis and the blood transfusion itself. The prevention and cure of Thalassemia lies in avoiding all kinds of suspected causes and changing the life style in accordance to the 'Living Water Therapy.'

# Disclaimer

1. Living Water Therapy for thalassemia is not approved by any government body. One may follow it in good faith, with a promise not to go for litigation under any circumstances.

2. Medicine/hospital related advise is entirely patients decision/call.

# CURE FOR BLOOD DISORDERS

## Thalassemia & Cancer

Dr. Biswaroop Roy Chowdhury

DIAMOND BOOKS

**India Office:**
**C/o India Book of Records**
B-121, 2nd Floor, Greenfields,
Faridabad -120003 (Haryana),
India
Ph.: +91-9312286540

**Malaysia Office:**
**C/o Bishwaroop International Healing & Research**
PT 573, Lot 15077 Jalan Tuanku
Munawir,
70000 Negeri Sembilan, Malaysia
Tel: +6012-2116089

**Vietnam Office:**
**C/o Vietnam Book of Records**
148 Hong Ha Street
9 Award, Phu Nhuan District,
Ho Chi Minh City, Vietnam
- Hotline: (+84) 903710505

**Switzerland Office:**
**C/o Nigel Kingsley**
Kraftwerkstr. 95, ch-5465, Mellikon,
Switzerland
Tel: 0041 79 222 2323

FOLLOW ME

**Facebook:** https://www.facebook.com/drbrc.official/
**Twitter:** https://twitter.com/drbrcofficial
**Bitchute:** https://www.bitchute.com/channel/drbiswarooproychowdhury/
**Instagram:** https://www.instagram.com/dr.biswarooproychowdhury/
**Telegram:** https://t.me/drbiswarooproychowdhury
**Email:** biswaroop@biswaroop.com
**Website:** www.biswaroop.com
**Video Channel:** www.coronakaal.tv

**Research :** Rachna Sharma
**Graphics Designer**: Shankar Singh Koranga, Prabha Shankar Sharma
**Copy Editor**: Divya Sharma
**Patient Mentoring & Counseling :** Dr. Namita Gupta (MBBS, MD)

Published by
**Diamond Pocket Books**
X-30, Okhla Industrial Area, New Delhi-110020
Ph: 011-40712100 email: sales@dpb.in website: www.diamondbook.in

# Dedication

Dedicated to my angel daughter Ivy,

loving wife Neerja

&

caring parents

Shri Bikash Roy Chowdhury

Shrimati Lila Roy Chowdhury

# CONTENTS

## SECTION - I



## SECTION - II

# SECTION -I

**Thalassemia, Sickle cell anemia, or various types and stages of Cancer, this section will help you understand various kinds of blood disorders beyond the conventionally accepted definition. From the consensus in medical science to the conspiracy of medical industry, this section will lead you to the potential solution and a permanent cure to end the incessant dependency on blood transfusion and the silent suffering of the patients.**

CHAPTER -1

# Filmy Director V/s Real life Doctors

★

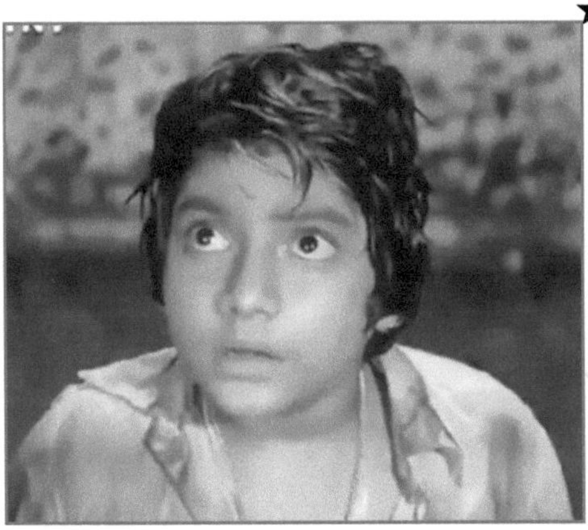

If you are of my age (by the way I am going to be 50 next year) you will certainly recognize this child. He appeared in more than 300 films in his career as a child artist. Whether it was Coolie, Shakti, Amar Akbar Anthony, or Daku Mangal Pandey, mostly in the first few minutes of the beginning of the film, the child suddenly transforms into an angry young man as a coolie, a smuggler, a don, or a dacoit. None of the viewers of the film bothers to know the in-between connection of the scenes. We as an audience understand that it is just how the movie has been scripted and is completely out of our jurisdiction. The film is merely for the sake of entertainment and we need not take it too seriously or even try to probe into the in-between scientific, logical connection or the proof of evidence.

---

★ To know more about the child, go to page no.149

However, this should not be our attitude when it is matter of life and death. Now look at another child's picture below.

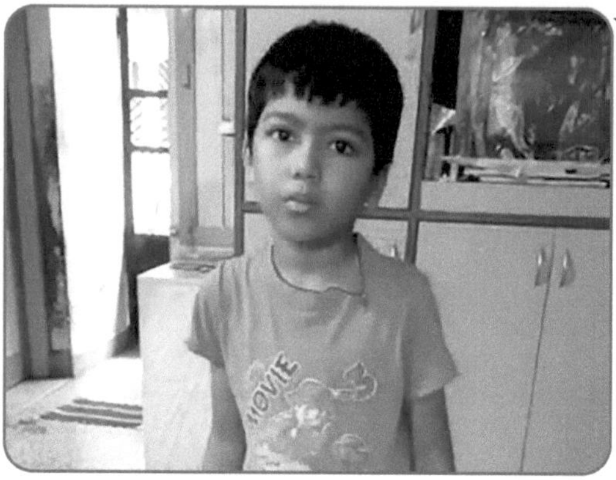
★★

Not out of any film but from a Gujrati family in Vadodara, this child's name is Hetkash Zanzrukiya and he had been healthy till he was 3 months old. Suddenly, one day just based on a blood test he was declared a so-called Thalassemia patient. Further, with no logic whatsoever, based on nothing but guess work, doctors declared his parents also thalassemia minor, meaning the parents are to be blamed for the present health status of the child. In turn, it means at least once or twice a month the child had to go for painful blood transfusion, depending on others' blood for his survival. By the time he reaches his 25 years, his chances of death will remain approximately 50% or by the time he will be say, of my age his chances of death will be nearly 100%. Also, all through his shortened life he will be mostly ill.

★★ To know more about the child, go to page no.83

**Mean age of Thalassemia patient is 23.81 years**

The survival rate of patients with beta-thalassemia major and intermedia and its trends in recent years in Iran

*Alireza Ansari-Moghaddam1 , Hossein Ali Adineh2 , Iraj Zareban3 , Mehdi Mohammadi1 , Mahtab Maghsoodlu4*

*1 Health Promotion Research Center, Zahedan University of Medical Sciences, Zahedan, Iran; 2 Department of Epidemiology and Biostatistics, Iranshahr University of Medical Sciences, Iranshahr, Iran; 3 Department of Health Education, Health Promotion Research Center, Zahedan University of Medical Sciences, Zahedan, Iran; 4 Research Center, Iran Blood Transfusion Organization, Tehran, Iran*

Take a moment now and just try to gather the emotional turmoil the parents must be going through. Often upon my interaction with such parents, they confess of even deciding to commit suicide.

After knowing the stories of hundreds of such parents, I don't have any doubt in stating that, getting one's child diagnosed or rather falsely labeled as thalassemic is the most painful emotional upheaval among all of grief and sadness.

Here to my understanding, the only cause of this human suffering is we as social animals are programmed to behave like the audience of a film that never doubts or questions the Doctors, assuming it is not your jurisdiction. At most you will take a 2nd or 3rd opinion from other doctors, who belong to the same fraternity. Hence, in all likelihoods, the reply will remain same or unchanged.

In order to understand the truth of the so called hereditary disease, let us take an example. Imagine that you live in a city where everyone uses a bicycle as a mode of transportation.One is allowed only to use a cycle as a vehicle for transportation. No other vehicle is allowed in that city.

Every 500 meters there is a provision of a cycle repair shop available for anyone who needs to get their cycle repaired. The uniqueness about these shops is that the mechanics employed there are all educated and have graduated with degrees in cycle repairing. Therefore, all the mechanics of these cycle repair shops adopt a corporate-style culture of formal dressing for work.

Now imagine one day, while riding your bicycle, your cycle chain comes off. You are stranded on the road and are forced to visit the nearest cycle repair shop for getting the problem fixed.The cycle mechanic decides to identify the root cause of the problem as per the protocol. He takes time to diagnose the cause with seemingly hi-fi diagnostic tools and apprises you after a long waiting period about his findings. He says he checked the cycle for a number of factors like velocity, air pressure, weight, etc. After careful inspection he has come to a conclusion saying there is no cure for the problem. The only available solution according to him is for you sit on the cycle which he will push in such a manner that it will take you at least to the next cycle repair shop. He asks you to get the same push service from the mechanic in the next shop as well so that you can move ahead and continue your journey. Following the pattern, as long as you want to use the cycle, you will need to employ this strategy of paying a cycle repair shop mechanic to push your cycle so that it reaches the nearby destination.

Surprised at this diagnosis, you take your cycle to a new cycle repair shop for a second opinion. You ask the next mechanic if the first diagnosis makes any sense to him. He too being educated similarly from the same college affirms that the diagnosis is 'on the dot'. He agrees that the only available solution to the chronic problem is that the cycle needs to be pushed from one workshop to the next for the rest of its life span. The cycle can no longer be ridden using the paddles.

As you must have tried using the paddles and failed at achieving a successful ride, you ascertain the diagnosis to be true and accept the fate of the bicycle.

You notice others too suffer a similar fate with their cycles on the road and join them in paying the cycle mechanics for every push to your cycle from one workshop to the next.

One fine day you encounter someone like me who asks you the reason for paying the cycle repair mechanic for pushing your cycle from one repair workshop to the next. He suggests that by merely lifting the cycle chain and fixing it on the gear, you will be able to use the paddles easily and ride the cycle yourself without the push each time. You won't even have to pay the cycle mechanic for the push every time you take your cycle out on the road.

However, in that city there is a law known as the 'Drug and Magic Remedy Act' which lays down the rules such that anybody who suggests the remedy to the cycle owners of fixing the chain to solve the problem will be taken into custody and sent to jail. As a consequence, anybody who knows the solution will obviously keep his mouth shut owing to the punishment of being jailed. However, if he is brave enough to help people out of their misery by telling them a simple way out, he will be put behind bars for violating the city regulations.

In other words, several seemingly difficult problems have surprisingly simple solutions. However, the problem is scaled-up inordinately instead and a business model is created around it.

The example shared above is in line with the so-called genetic disorder Thalassemia. Rather, it is much more than that. Let me elucidate it further.

Consider a situation which actually might have happened with some of us. While you are travelling on a highway sometimes you realize your car's tyre has been punctured. Just then you notice you are very close to a puncture repair shop. You thank your stars at the coincidence of the tyre getting punctured right near a puncture repair shop.

What you didn't know that the puncture was a part of a strategy. A number of nails were thrown on the road in order to puncture the tyres of the vehicles passing through. The nails were thrown with an estimate of how long will it take for the drivers to realize that their vehicle's tyre has punctured. So within a couple of kilometres, the scrupulous individuals set up their puncture repair shops.

This is the same modus operendi in case of Thalassemia as well. In reality, Thalassemia was never a disease and none of the humans ever contract this disease. However, it is important to understand the truth behind the Thalassemia scam. In order to do so, let us take a real life example of a patient, Hetkash.

Hetkash was one day suddenly diagnosed with Thalassemia. How did he come to know this? It was through the reports of a random test conducted by him. As his haemoglobin was low in the reports, he was recommended blood transfusion as the only solution to the problem.

While on the one hand, blood transfusion is recommended in order to increase the haemoglobin in the patient's body, the side-effect of this procedure itself decreases the haemoglobin count of the patient's body.

Medically, this is known as 'Delayed Haemolytic Transfusion Reaction' (DHTR).

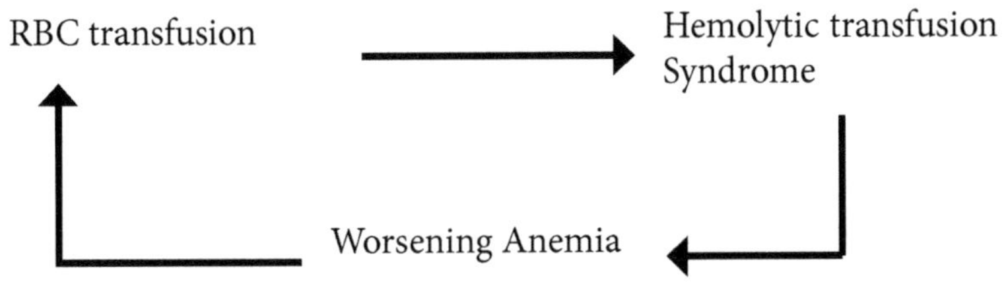


*Leung J, Weiskopf RB, Feiner J, et al. Electrocardiographic STsegment changes during acute, severe isovolemic hemodilution in humans. Anesthesiology. 2000;93:1004-10*

When blood transfusion is conducted on a patient, it can be considered similar to a procedure for organ transplant. Initially, the patient's body considers the donated organ as a foreign body and rejects it. As part of the basic nature of the body, it attacks the donated organ considering it as an external agent.

**Blood transfusion can be viewed as an organ transplant with known complexities and risks**

*Shander A. Emerging risks and outcomes of blood transfusion in surgery. Semin Hematol 2004; 41: 117–24*

Similarly, during the process of blood transfusion, the patient's body for most of the patients, considers the external blood as a foreign body and generates antibodies in the system in order to attack the transfused blood protein. These antibodies start destroying the Red

Blood Cells of its own body. This is known as Delayed Haemolytic Transfusion Reaction.

**Risks of allogeneic blood transfusion should be viewed in the context of the assertion that efficacy of RBC transfusions in improving patient outcomes is largely unestablished. Using evidence from published literature, a panel of clinicians recently rated allogeneic blood transfusions unlikely or uncertain to improve patient outcomes in the vast majority of common hypothetical clinical scenarios in which blood transfusions are commonplace.**

*Shander A, Fink A, Javidroozi M, et al. Appropriateness of allogeneic red blood cell transfusion: the international consensus conference on transfusion outcomes. Transfus Med Rev 2011; 25: 232–46*

It is important to note, there are several factors that may lead to a decrease in haemoglobin in an individual's body. For instance, during fever a patient's haemoglobin mostly decreases by two to four grams/dl. When the patient recovers, the haemoglobin levels also increase back to the original count.

**Hemoglobin Levels Vary in Infants in Relation in Occurrence of Influenza Virus Infections.**

*Tom Adamkiewicz, Omolaya Dada, Patrick O'Neil, Erica Wong, McKinley Tran; Blood 2019; 134 (Supplement_1): 4813.*

During high body temperature, when a patient takes any antipyretic medication like a paracetamol, this too results in a severe decrease in haemoglobin count in the body.

**Antipyretic Therapy: Physiologic Rationale, Diagnostic Implications, and Clinical Consequences.**

*Plaisance KI, Mackowiak PA. Arch Intern Med. 2000;160(4):449–456. doi:10.1001/archinte.160.4.449*

In cases when a patient is identified as a so- called Thalassemia patient and blood transfusion is recommended as a course of treatment for increasing the haemoglobin range in the body, the blood transfusion itself causes damage to the body and results in the reduction of haemoglobin in the patient's body. Within two to four weeks of the transfusion, the haemoglobin count reduces and this time the reason for reduction is not any of the genetic factors or having anything to do with the child's health. Instead, it is due to the side-effect of the blood transfusion. At that point, the doctor must appraise the patient about the actual reason of the decrease of the haemoglobin level. It can be due to fever where it is natural to see a decrease in haemoglobin levels; or perhaps, it was due to the medication given to the patient, which is also a very natural phenomenon in general; or maybe the damage in the body was due to the blood transfusion procedure.

**Treatment with erythropoiesis stimulating agents (ESAs) agents comes with risks of its own and has been linked to increased risk of mortality and cardiovascular events**
**Thus, whether the outcomes seen in anaemic patients are related to anaemia or treatment with ESAs is unclear.**

*Singh AK. What is causing the mortality in treating the anaemia of chronic kidney disease: erythropoietin dose or hemoglobin level? CurrOpin Nephrol Hypertens 2010; 19: 420–4*

However, instead of sharing the actual reason for the decrease in the haemoglobin levels in the patient, doctors have created a new terminology as a reason behind it. They say, the decrease in haemoglobin levels is due to a genetic reason and put the blame on the parents of the patient. It can therefore, be inferred that the patient is suffering with low haemoglobin count because of the parents. However, it must be noted that the actual fault lies with the doctors and their treatment protocols.

There are several factors that can be instrumental in getting a child falsely diagnosed as a patient of Thalassemia. One of most widespread factor is vaccination.

**One case report found that a child developed aplastic anaemia three weeks after receiving the chickenpox vaccine. The authors concluded that "paediatricians should be aware of this severe although rare" side-effect of the vaccine.**

*Angelini et. al, 2009*

**Influenza (flu) vaccine: The flu vaccine has been known to cause relapses in people who previously suffered from aplastic anaemia.**

*Hendry et. al, 2002*

It has been observed that post vaccinations, a large majority of children fall prey to health issues like Thalassemia, Type 1 Diabetes, or ADHD. As in case of Diabetes, children experience a temporary increase in blood sugar levels in their bodies while in Thalassemia, a temporary decrease in haemoglobin is observed. Now by taking advantage of this unfortunate phase in the lives of children, instead of giving their parents the right diagnosis and guidance, doctors make efforts to make the child drug dependent and hospital dependent for life.

In case of Type 1 Diabetes, the doctors should have advised parents to feed the child with lots of fruits and vegetables and to avoid any animal food. In no time the child's blood sugar would have come back to the normal level. Instead, they give insulin injections and advise the parents to increase the intake of animal protein for the child. In other words, the doctors play a major role in ensuring the suffering of the children.

In line with our initial bicycle example, when parents visit a different doctor for a second opinion, the second doctor also having studied the same pattern of education and being a part of the same white coat gang, provides the same diagnosis and recommends the same solution to the parents.

When parents listen to the same pattern of problem and solution from various doctors, they are convinced that their child's suffering actually is their own fault which they have genetically passed on to the child. In this manner, this business of disease mongering thrives.

## Case Study – Reversal of Type 1 Diabetes Using Plant Based Diet

***Dr. Biswaroop Roy Chowdhury***

*Journal of the Science of Healing Outcomes, Jan 2021 (Vol 13, No. 50)*

It is essential to remember that hospitals and pharmaceutical companies can never benefit from a healthy individual. The same is true with a dead person. Business can only be generated from those individuals who are alive along with some disease or health condition Only such individuals can fuel the pharmaceutical business across the world. Therefore, the medical network is created in such a manner that not only one is alive, but also consistently maintains ill-health. Their dependence on drugs and medications continues for a lifetime. As in case of Type 1Diabetes, the pharmaceutical profits increase every time a patient buys insulin injections. Similarly, in case of Thalassemia, where even if a patient undergoes free blood transfusion as part of a Government scheme, the pharmaceutical companies make profit through the taxpayer's money. This way ultimately everything goes from your own pockets to the pharmaceutical companies.

It is interesting to note that the pharmaceutical industry has been known for making highest donations to political parties. When these political parties come to power, it becomes their moral responsibility to promote the industry that has been instrumental in their winning the elections and coming to power. In order to continue with the profitable existence of this pharmaceutical industry, all evidences that prove the real reason behind the diagnosis of the so-called Thalassemia or Type 1 Diabetes diseases are hidden from the general masses. The temporary reduction in haemoglobin in case of Thalassemia or the temporary increase in blood sugar in case of Type 1 Diabetes is declared as permanent and chronic diseases when in fact, these health conditions can be reversed. However, the evidences are never allowed to come in the main stream.

Hundreds of Diabetes Type 1 patients could free themselves of insulin once they adopted my recommended DIP Diet and the first 40 blood transfusion patients (thalassemic) since July 2022 could free themselves of blood transfusion and the dependency on drugs once they started following my recommended 'The Living Water Therapy' (read more about it in the next chapter). This is a proof that these disorders are not genetic disorders rather, suspected side-effect of vaccine, drug administration, or just a wrong diagnosis followed by the recommendation of regular dependency on blood transfusion leading to more widespread damage to the body. Had the diseases really been genetic disorders, it would not have been possible to reverse the health condition back to normal state.

CHAPTER -2

# Thalassemia Cure

By now you must have understood that blood transfusion is not a solution or a cure for thalassemia. Instead, getting blood transfusion done is like falling in a trap. If you ask any doctor if there exists a cure for Thalassemia, you will get a response that the only solution is a bone-marrow transplant. However, the on-ground reality is that 40% of the children who get a bone-marrow transplant are unable to survive beyond one year. On an average, it has been observed all those children who have undergone a bone-marrow transplant in childhood do not have a lifespan beyond 15 years of age.

Survival Statistics by Year of Bone Marrow Transplant Patients

| **Days** | **Years** | **Alive at Year Start** |
|---|---|---|
| 1096-1460 | 3-4 | 587 |
| 1461-1825 | 4-5 | 484 |
| 2191-2555 | 6-7 | 368 |
| 2556-2920 | 7-8 | 318 |
| 2921-3285 | 8-9 | 277 |
| 3286-3650 | 9-10 | 240 |
| 3651-4015 | 10-11 | 205 |
| 4016-4380 | 11-12 | 171 |
| 4381-4745 | 12-13 | 143 |
| 4746-5110 | 13-14 | 118 |
| 5111-5475 | 14-15 | 99 |

**Long-Term Survival after Blood and Marrow Transplantation: Comparison with an Age- and Gender-Matched Normative Population**
*Biology of Blood and Marrow Transplantation 12:430-437 (2006)*
*2006 American Society for Blood and Marrow Transplantation*
*1083-8791/06/1204-0006$32.00/0 doi:10.1016/j.bbmt.2005.12.026*

Moreover, not only do the parents bear a cost of Rs 25 to Rs 30 lakhs towards this costly treatment, it is also an excruciatingly painful and a dangerous process, both for the donor as well as a patient.

A bone-marrow transplant reduces the lifespan of a Thalassemia patient. As a serious side-effect of the procedure, it can also cause paralysis or even death for the healthy person who donates his bone marrow towards the procedure. There are several other side- effects of the transplant that are never even discussed, for instance, insomnia, experiencing weakness for a prolonged period of time, apart from pain in bones and the body for a prolonged period of time. It can easily be inferred, for the pharmaceutical industry, a patient of blood transfusion is like the golden goose who lays a golden egg on regular intervals.

The inordinate greed can lead the owner to kill the goose in order to take all the golden eggs at once. Similarly, a bone marrow transplant is a way in which the patient is required to pay Rs 25 lakhs to Rs 30 lakhs towards the procedure despite the knowledge that the transplant will only have an adverse effect on the patient and further damage his system. Notwithstanding, the bone marrow transplant poses a grave threat to the lives of both the patient as well as the bone marrow donor.

It is critical to understand the ways in which we can take preventive measures towards the situation. As much as I understand in view of my patients' histories, there is a occurrence of fever. The parents often share they took their child to a doctor for the treatment of fever. When the health of the child kept deteriorating, the doctor recommended some tests to be conducted on the child. Thereafter, based on the reports the doctor declared their child as a Thalassemia patient. When the parents, enquire how all of a sudden their child has been diagnosed with Thalassemia, the doctors put that blame on the parents saying Thalassemia is a genetic condition that comes to the child from his parents. The doctors explain that the child inherits a faulty gene from his parents which causes him to suffer from Thalassemia, making parents responsible for the child's health condition.

By now you must have understood that Thalassemia is not a genetic disorder. In the initial stages, it can be mentioned as anemia or having low hemoglobin count in the body. When anybody, especially a child, has fever then throughout the duration of the fever the hemoglobin levels of the child fall by a few counts. For instance if the normal hemoglobin count of the healthy child is 12 then during fever, his count can fall down to 9 or even lower counts.

**Diarrhea and fever as risk factors for anemia among children under age five living in urban slum areas of Indonesia**

*International Journal of Infectious Diseases, Volume 12, Issue 1,2008, Richard D. Semba, Saskia de Pee, Michelle O. Ricks, Mayang Sari, Martin W. Bloem*

However, if the child is given heavy doses of antibiotic and antipyretic medicines in the name of treatment then as a side-effect of the medication the child's hemoglobin drops in the body. Low hemoglobin further deteriorates the health of the child and the doctor declares him as a patient of Thalassemia.

You learned in the first chapter, ways in which you are liable to fall in the trap and the number of factors that almost breadcrumb their way to the lifelong trap of suffering with Thalassemia. The more prevalent and frequent of these factors is fever which occurs most frequently in children.

Fever itself is not a trigger to create a permanent damage to the body. Fever leads to your decision to take antipyretic, antibiotic, and other medicines and together this causes damage. And when your child is diagnosed with anemia (or they call it thalassemia) and opt for blood transfusion, you cause more intense damage to the child's body. The child becomes a slave to the medical industry for life and becomes transfusion dependent.

Through this book I would like to advise all parents never to give antibiotic or antipyretic medicines to your child whenever he has fever or flu-like symptoms. Instead of drugs, you must adopt a three-step flu diet along with the heat protocol. We administer this diet to all of our patients, whether they visit our hospital or are connected with us virtually.

**To learn The Heat Protocol and 3- Step Flu diet read :**

***Download the book from www.biswaroop.com/ebooks***

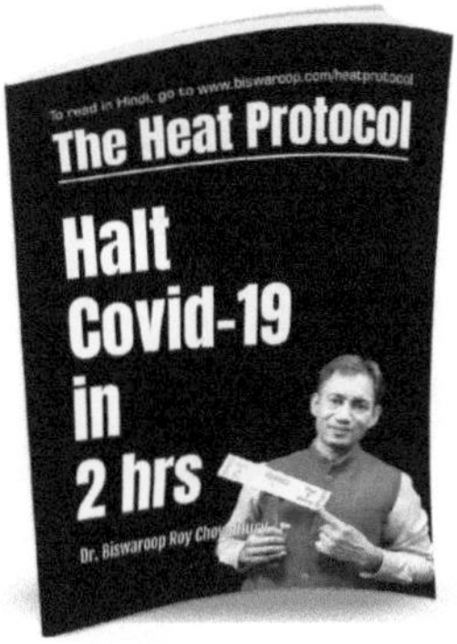

To understand the procedure of the same you can visit the above web link and read a book which elaborates the process simply and in easy steps. You can also watch a small video that takes you through the entire process easily. Within 15 minutes you can become a master of heat protocol and along with the three-step flu diet you can magically control all symptoms of flu and ease your fever. By following the procedures accurately, you will also be successfully able to avoid getting into the clutches of the pharmaceutical industry.

This is a simple precautionary way to avoid falling in the trap of blood transfusion Industry. But what can you do if you are already a declared thalessemia patient and also undergo blood transfusion therapy on a regular basis? In such a situation, I recommend one solution which I call the Living Water Therapy. When patients who are dependent on blood transfusion from one to even five times a month, adopt the Living Water Therapy, their chances of transfusion become almost negligible.

So let us now understand the most important part of the book where we learn the Living Water Therapy. I hope after adopting this therapy in your own lives, you will share its benefits with your loved ones and with those in need. Wherever possible, you will share the Living Water Therapy technique far and wide for the goodness of humanity.

You must understand no matter how much one experiences deterioration in his health, no matter how low his hemoglobin drops, there are certain life style modifications and factors with the help of which he can increase his hemoglobin levels in a natural way. The health condition can always be reversed to a stable condition.

The easiest way to understand this is by the way of the following image of spring water.

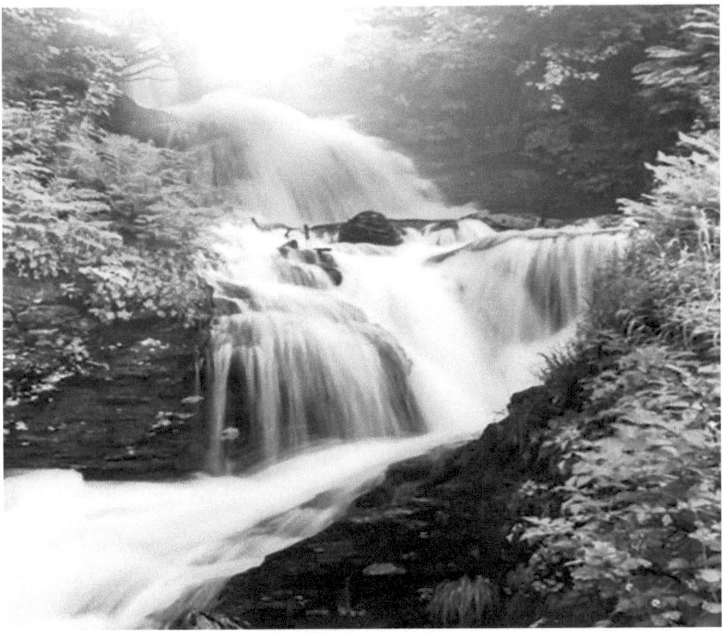

Spring water is not merely water, but it is 'Amrit' or the elixir of life.

When you drink this spring-water you can claim to have found the solution. In case you are looking for a single line cure for Thalassemia, then whichever part of the world you live, simply pack your bags and fly to a place with an easy access to spring water and make it your home. Whenever you feel thirsty, make sure you drink water out of this spring. Look for fruits and vegetables that grow around this spring and you can consume them in raw form for best results. The day you are able to successfully lead this kind of lifestyle, you can consider yourself cured or at least are on your way to better health. Spend time as much time around the spring water as possible. Walk barefoot in the sunlight on the natural grass that surrounds the spring, taking in fresh air with each step. This is the complete solution, which we call the Living Water Therapy. This spring water is referred to as the living water while the water you consume on a daily basis filtering through an RO water purifier is nothing but dead water.

The RO filter in your household in reality is not a water purifier but a slow poisoning mechanism. The water filtered through an RO slowly and gradually mingles poison in our system and don't realize when or how our health deteriorates.

Simply put, the water from an RO filter is demineralized water. Whether or not it removes bacteria viruses and harmful chemicals from the water, it definitely removes the most essential part of water by demineralizing the water and ripping it off all the nutrients. You consume this demineralized water thinking it to be a purified water. If the water contained all the essential minerals it would positively impact your body by letting the body absorb all the nutrients. This RO filter water instead strips off minerals from the body and pushes whatever minerals are present in the body out of the system through urine.

Your body consistently becomes demineralized by drinking water from an RO filter. Therefore, RO water is also a major contributor to promoting various modern day diseases, not just blood disorders. With immediate effect all RO filter users must uninstall and throw away filters from our homes and offices. In addition, one must remove the use of bottled water from our lives and replace it with living water.

**National Green Tribunal has issues a ban on the use of Reverse Osmosis (RO) water purifiers in India from December 2020 onwards.**

You may think I am asking you to pack up all your belongings, sell your homes and cars etc, and shift to the Himalayas or the mountain regions near spring water. This is definitely not the case. It is a mere option for those who can adopt this life. I understand with the kind of lifestyle and daily activities we indulge in, it is impossible to even fathom moving away from our present day lives and involvements. Unfortunately, we are not even able to take out enough time from our schedules to visit such places for a few days, let alone shift base altogether.

We have tied ourselves to this modern lifestyle where we don't have the freedom to control our own lives. Our lives are governed by someone else and we are mere bonded laborers and followers who complete one activity after another as per orders, making our own lives a burden to carry rather than an emancipated individual who has complete control over his life's decisions.

Keeping this in perspective, let me now give you a practical alternative which can easily be adopted at home. I have been successfully imparting this knowledge to all my patients, whether they live in the city or rural areas of our country and whatever be their financial status in society. I call it the three-pot water system. You must have definitely seen it before or heard of it previously in life. You are simply unaware of its importance in our lives and the miraculous benefits we can get from this three-pot water system. All you have to do is to bring home three earthen pots and create the system by yourself and reap unlimited benefits thereafter.

The procedure to create the three-pot system is as follows:

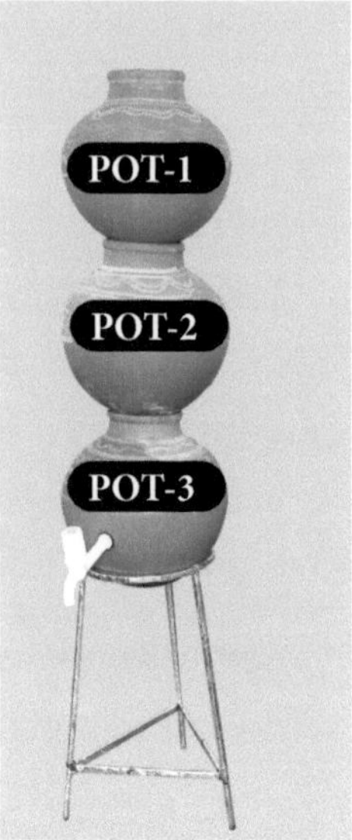


## Step 1 - Living water therapy

The first step is creating the three pot system at home and drinking living water from this system every time you need to use water all through the day. It must be noted no other source of water must be used as part of the therapy.

## Procedure to prepare 3 Pot System

**Step1: Arrange mineral stones, small marbles, fine-grained stones, sand, wood charcoal.**

**Step2:** Wash all the above-mentioned ingredients one by one separately in buckets thoroughly 4 to 5 times.

**Step 3:** Arrange drumstick / moringa seeds and grind them into a fine powder.

**Step 4:** Arrange a Copper plate.

**Step 5:** Arrange 3 pots as shown in the picture above. One of the pot should have a tap fitted in it.

**Step 6:** At the base of pot 1 which is placed on the top, make a few small holes to create a sieve-like effect.

The same will be repeated for pot 2 (placed in the middle).

**Step 7:** Put small stones, marbles and fine-grained stones in layers one by one on top 2 pots.

**Step 8:** Then add sand, and on the topmost, layer add the wood charcoal.

Fill the pots up to half of their capacity.

**Step 9:** In pot 3 put drumstick/ moringa seed powder and a copper plate.

**Step 10:** Now add fresh tap water or RO water in pot 1 which is on the top. Fill it up to the brim.

Wait for 8-9hrs. The water from the top most pot will filter down to the second (middle pot) and then finally into the lowermost pot.

The water collected in Pot 3 is the living water.

## Xylem Water Filter

Plant xylem tissue, a process material that conducts tissue in the plants, with the pores size typically from few nanometers to a maximum of around 500mm ideal for filtering out pathogen. The safest way to get rid of bacteria from the water is by fitting xylem filter at the bottom of the 2nd pot.

**Steps for making xylem filter:**

1. Peel the bark (at least 1 cm in diameter) of any coniferous tree.
2. Cut the piece in about 1cm length.
3. Fasten it into the tube with the help of fastener.
4. Fit the piece at the bottom of the 2nd pot.

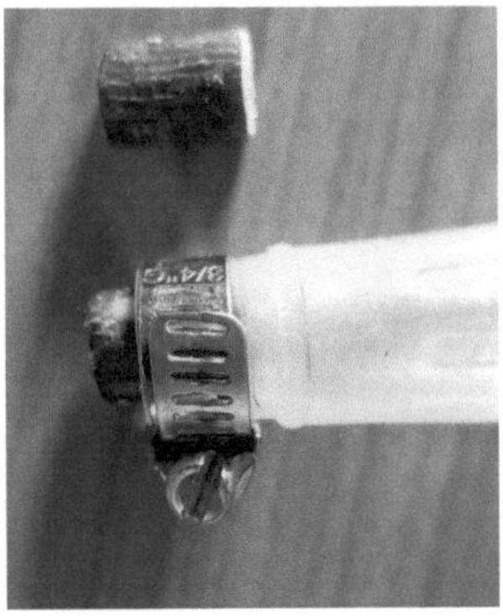

| **Water Filtration Using Plant Xylem.** |
| --- |
| *Boutilier MSH, Lee J, Chambers V, Venkatesh V, Karnik R (2014) PLoS ONE 9(2): e89934. https://doi.org/10.1371/journal.pone.0089934* |

## Step 2 – Living food therapy

As part of this step you must consume only that food which contains living water in it.

For instance, if we take tomato, you will be surprised to know that it contains 96% water and the remaining 4% contains other nutrients. So when you consume tomatoes, you are inadvertently consuming 96% living water in the process. So the water contained in a tomato is known as living water. In fact, all the fruits and vegetables contain 70% to 90% of living water in them.

All you need to do is to consume fruits and raw vegetables as part of your diet. You must ensure that at least 90% of your diet contains raw fruits and vegetables. Including them in your meals is an excellent way to improve your health.

Your breakfast can be consuming fruits as per your appetite and hunger. Choose three to four types of fruits of your choice and consume them in proportion to your weight.

For instance, if your weight is 70 kg, then take a minimum of 70 x 10= 700 grams fruits for breakfast. Please make sure that the fruits are taken before 12:00 Noon.

In case of a child below 10 years of age, you must double the quantity. For example,

if the weight of the child is 30 kg and age is below 8 years, then the calculation for quantity of fruits will be as follows:

30 x 20=600 grams of fruits for breakfast before noon.

This completes the first part of the Living water food therapy.

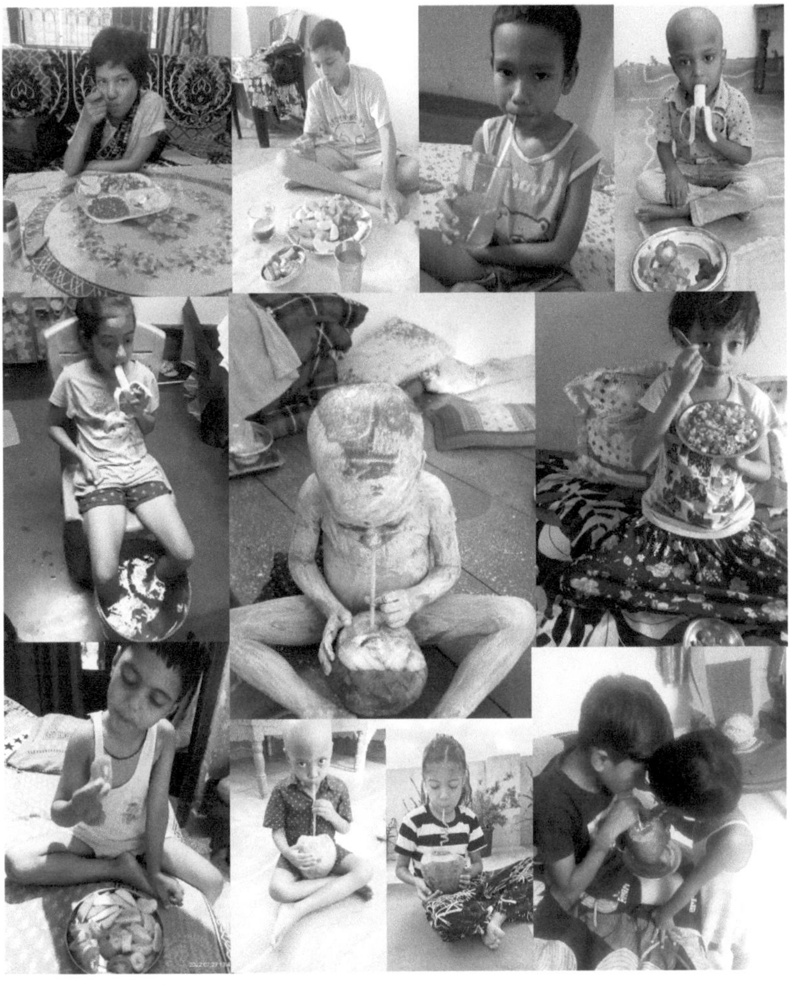

The second part includes the first meal of the day which we consume as lunch. Here one must consume steamed and raw vegetable lunch. You can again take between three to four kinds of vegetables which you can have raw, steamed, or a little boiled.

For instance, you have a range of vegetables to choose from like radish, cucumber, tomato, peas, spinach, all kinds of capsicum, etc. You can choose the vegetables of your preference and add them to your diet for lunch. While most of them can be consumed raw, you can steam or boil vegetables like broccoli, cauliflower, ladyfinger etc.

You can be creative and have three to four types of vegetables of your choice for lunch and have delicious meals every day. For some people, eating steamed or raw vegetables will be an acquired taste which over a period of time will accustom to your palate and you will not only start enjoying it, but also see visible results in form of good health.

It is critical to understand this diet will be instrumental in making you blood transfusion-free and Thalassemia-free over a period of time. You must consume as much as is enough to fill your stomach.

The measure can be determined for an individual by using the same formula. If for instance, you are 70kg in weight then your lunch diet can be based on the following formula:

70x10=700 grams of raw, steamed, or boiled vegetables in a combination for lunch.

Now let us take a look at what to have for dinner for a healthy and disease-free body. Our dinner must be consumed before 7:00 P.M. every day. Here too, we must first take our salad comprising raw, steamed, or boiled vegetables.

Even if you are not able to consume, say, 700 grams as per the example taken above, our effort should be to at least have enough to fill your stomach. For the main course, you have a leniency of having slightly cooked food. However, dinner must not include any kind of grains. Options like wheat, rice, millets must not be consumed for dinner. While these are not harmful foods it is seen to have an adverse auto-immune reaction in some children by way of destroying the red blood cells of our body causing our immunity to dip further down.

This tendency of the body to react to grains may be a result of vaccinations, or the consumption of drugs and medications, or some other unknown reason that is still a mystery to the world. Since this is a tendency observed after the consumption of grains, animal proteins, and animal food, I strongly recommend my patients to remove all kinds of dairy products, animal food, packaged food, and grains from our diet at all cost. We must make a conscious effort in understanding the ill-effects these products have on our bodies and the ways in which we suffer after consuming them. We must therefore, remove them from our diet altogether.

Let us take an example to understand this better. Consider some kerosene has accidentally fallen on the ground. Now even the smallest of sparks is enough to set the kerosene on fire leading to a grave situation. On the other hand, if the floor is dry and we create a spark or even fire and throw it on the ground, we will not see it spreading unduly all across the floor. As the floor is dry, it will help in extinguishing the fire instead of spreading it any further. It is important to understand that the spread or extinguishing of fire is dependent on the medium it uses. Similarly, if the children are likely to develop an auto-immune reaction after consuming animal based foods and grains, especially when they have been on a blood transfusion procedure for an elongated period of time, they must completely abstain from including them in their diet. This is because animal food and grains are known to trigger auto-immune reaction in children diagnosed with low hemoglobin or high blood sugar repeatedly.

As far as cooked food is concerned, you can choose to cook lentils, beans like rajma, or even vegetables and consume them as per your appetite and desire.

An important component of the living water food is the Green and Red Juice. Using a cold pressed juicer you can prepare one glass of juice of any green leafy vegetables of your choice. The chlorophyll in the leaves which gives the color green has a very similar structure to that of hemoglobin. The center of hemoglobin contains Iron while the center of chlorophyll contains Magnesium. This is the reason why chlorophyll can also be called Green Blood and this is how it is addressed as in the scientific community.

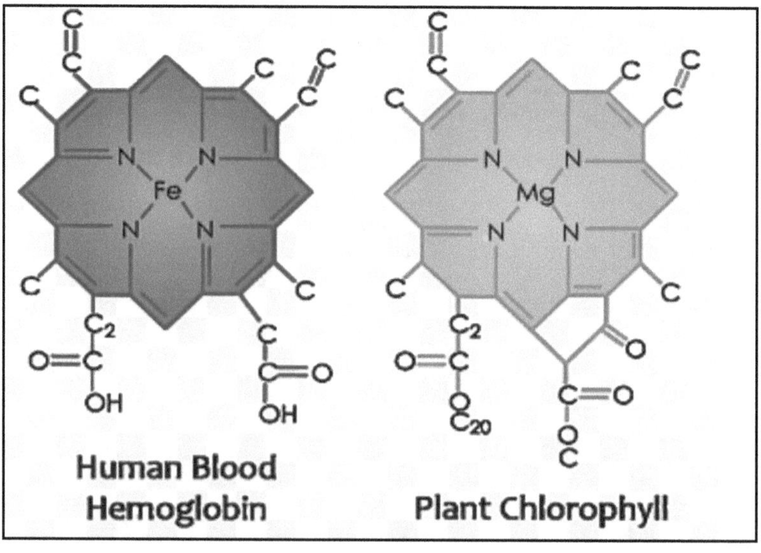

Therefore, it is recommended to consume a glass of green or red juice on a daily basis. You can also alternate the red and green juices in your diet. So while green juice is made from green leafy vegetables, red juice can be made using red vegetables. These can include tomatoes or beetroot made from a cold press juicer.

You can also use a combination of green and red juices in your diet. So for example, you can make a glass of juice using green leafy vegetables, tomatoes, and beetroot and include it as part of your meals. Apart from this you can also include sprouts in your diet.

## Step 3 – Grounding

Here it is recommended to be in constant touch with the ground beneath us. Humans are the only species on the planet which wears footwear to walk on the ground. This is the reason human beings are unable to connect themselves to the earth through the electromagnetic field. As a result, humans have to undergo a number of unforeseen

diseases and maladies in life.

I therefore, recommend to devote at least 15 minutes of earthing on a daily basis.

For this you must be barefoot and walk or play on the grass or in mud. Whatever activity you choose, make sure you are associated with the earth directly for at least some time during the day on a regular basis or as much as you can. This process is known as grounding.

**Grounding reduces RBC aggregation, increases the surface charge on it and reduces the blood viscosity**

*Chevalier G, Sinatra ST, Oschman JL, Delany RM. Earthing (grounding) the human body reduces blood viscosity-a major factor in cardiovascular disease. J Altern Complement Med. 2013 Feb;19(2):102-10. doi: 10.1089/acm.2011.0820. Epub 2012 Jul 3.*

**Picture of children on bushes, playing barefoot and walking barefoot on ground or in rain**

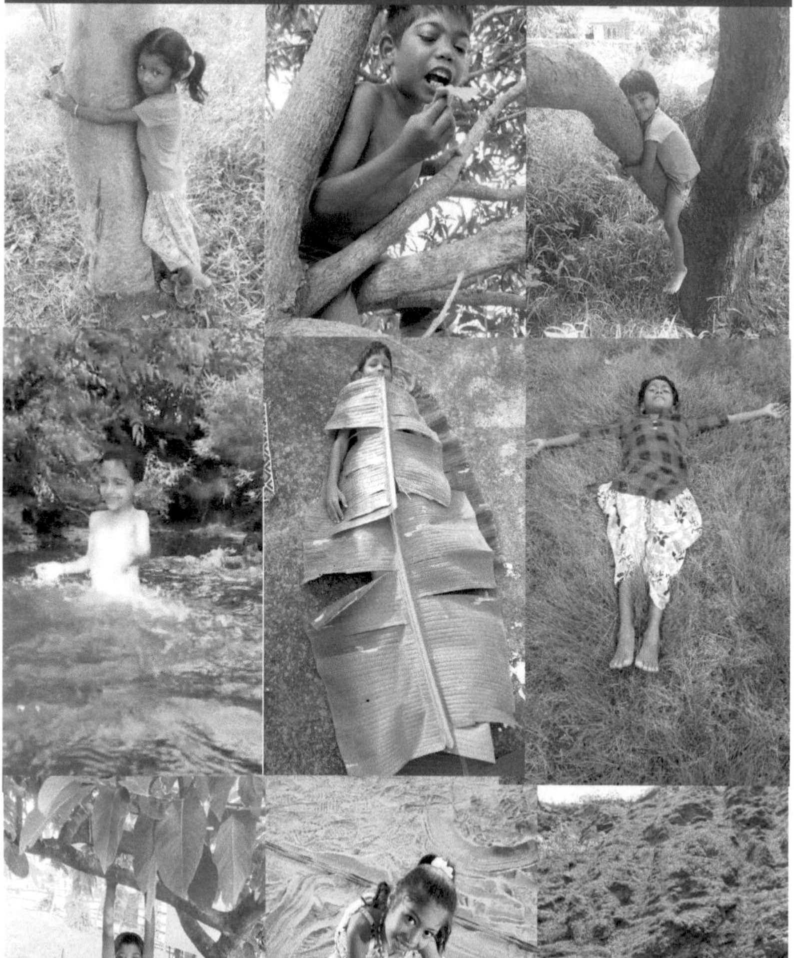

In addition, whenever it rains, make the most of it and soak yourself in rain. You can play in the rain or take a walk, or simply stand and enjoy the process of getting wet with rain water. These days modern day parents keep their children away from getting wet in direct rain. They scare the children away from the rains as if it is a rainfall of bullets instead of pure water.

If you aim for complete health for your body and a bright and clear skin devoid of any skin conditions then you must make efforts to get closer to Nature. The best way to be one with Nature is by grounding yourself and walking barefoot, being open to rain, etc. As you can see in this image, the children are joyfully grounding themselves by wrapping their hands around trees, climbing trees, and enjoying rain water. We must endeavor to include these as part of our lives on a regular basis for a complete holistic development and good health.

## Step 4 – Physical Activity

**An intensified training schedule in recreational male runners is associated with increases in erythropoiesis and inflammation and a net reduction in plasma hepcidin mild. The net effect is to decrease hepcidin concentrations and to tend to increase oral iron absorption.**

*Am J Clin Nutr2018;108:1324–1333.*

Remember to include physical activity of any kind as part of your daily regime. It can be playing sports, running, or any activity where your breathing increases must be a part of your daily life. An increase in the breathing rate directly increases the hemoglobin in your body and increases the RBC levels in your system.

**Picture of kids doing yoga /upside down etc**

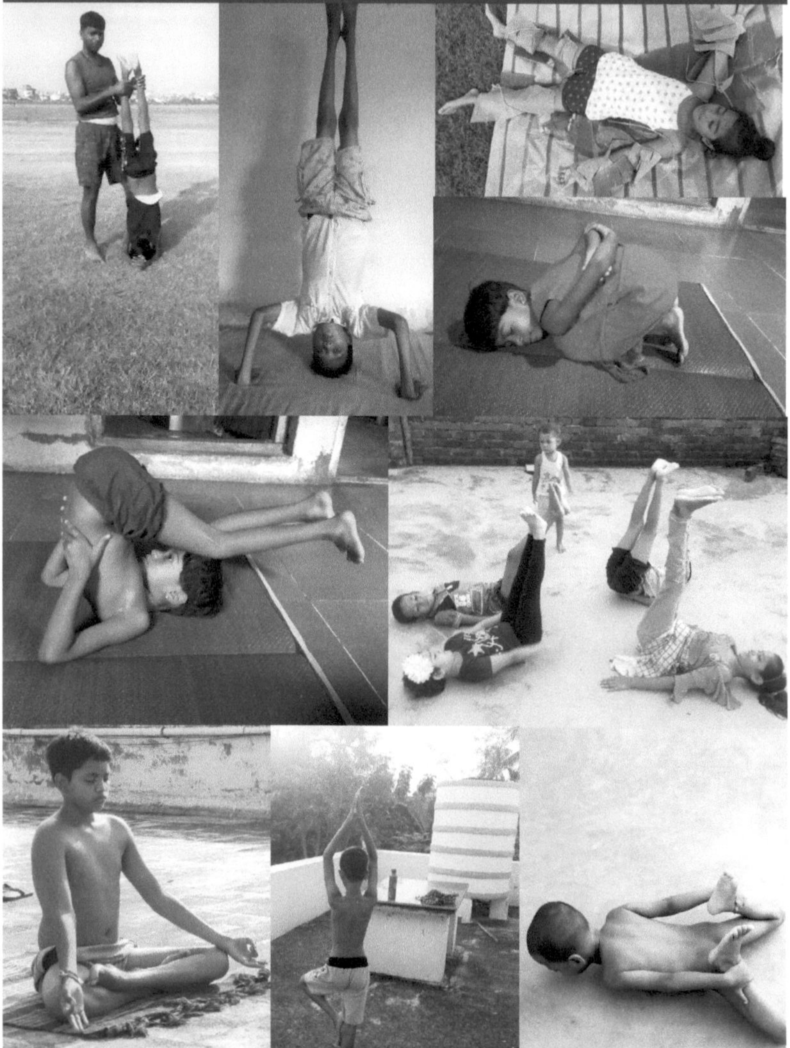

I have observed our modern public school education system gives little importance to playing, physical activities, or being out in the sun. As a result it has little precedence in the daily time table is given to physical activity in schools. Also, it is these children who are sheltered from the sun and physical activities who fall ill more frequently. Therefore, you must ensure to you include rigorous exercise and physical activity on a daily basis in your lives. A number of activities can be included in these such as playing football, dancing, spending time on swings, being out in the open during the morning or evening sun. You can choose an activity you enjoy the most, ensuring rigorous exercise and some quality time outside in the open, under the sun.

## Step 5- Lower Limb/ Upto neck Hot Water Immersion

This is an extremely important step as part of the treatment. One must include the lower limb hot water immersion therapy twice a day for at least 30 minutes each.

This is known to increase the iron absorption in the body. In addition, it increases the hemoglobin in the body along with increasing the production of Red Blood Cells in the body. This is a very powerful tool to repair and reverse the damages in the body which are a result of blood transfusion.

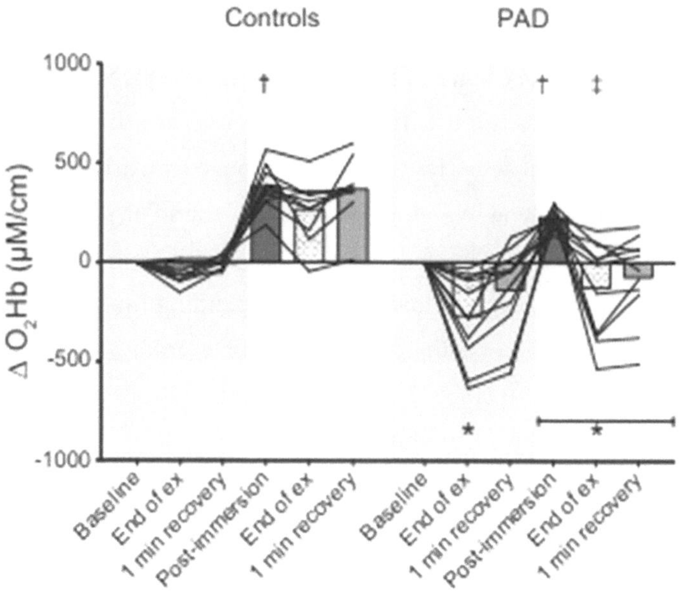


**Changes in muscle hemoglobin variables in response to lower-limb hot water immersion in the Control and PAD Group**
**The gray background indicates pre immersion, and the white background indicates post immersion.**

*AJP-RegulIntegr Comp Physiol • doi:10.1152/ajpregu.00404.2016 • www.ajpregu.org Downloaded from journals.physiology.org/journal/ajpregu (103.046.238.178) on August 17, 2022*

Normally, we provide this treatment to our patients of end-stage kidney failure. 70% of our patients at our HIIMS hospital are those who are on Dialysis and are recommended for a kidney transplant. As part of their treatment we give them the hot water immersion therapy where we take water at 40 degrees temperature and make the patient sit neck deep immersed in water.

**As shown in the images below, kids enjoying Hot Water Immersion**

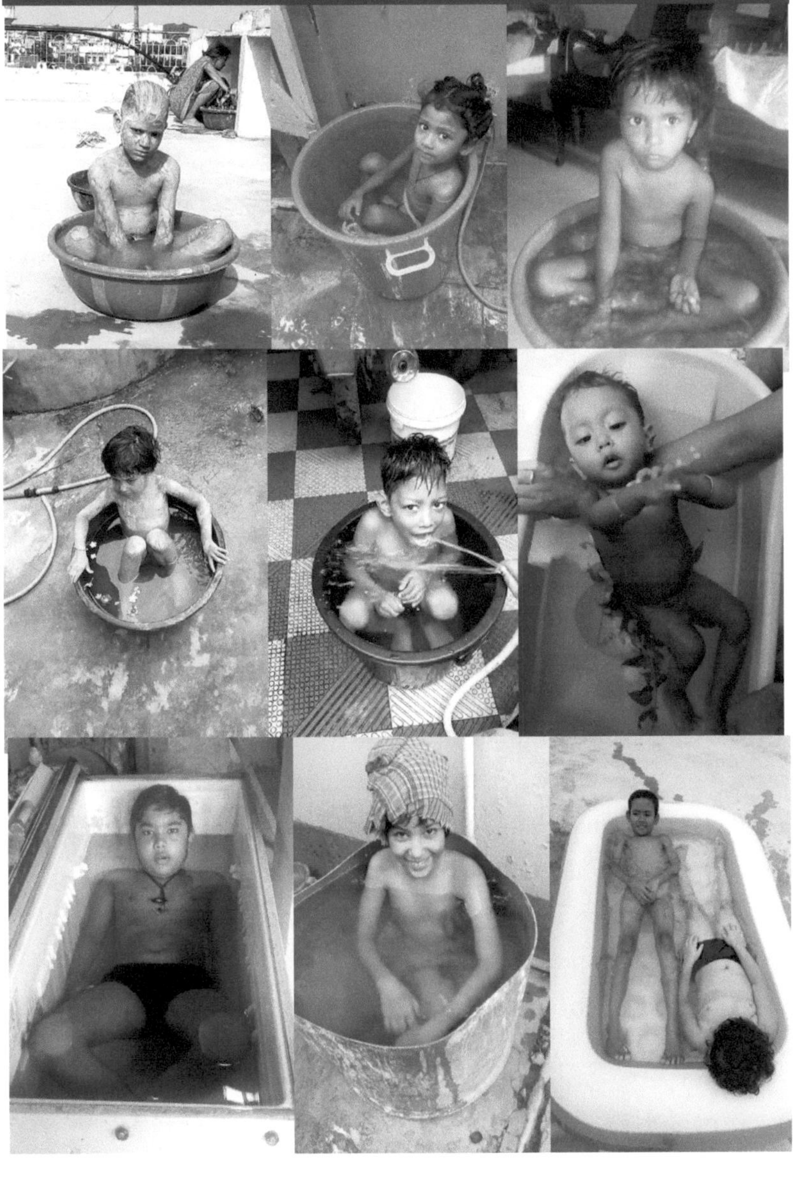

With regular therapy, we have been successful in making the patient free from the dependency on dialysis.

In case of a patient of Thalassemia, it is not necessary to sit neck deep in hot water.

Instead, the patient can suffice if they sit with their lower limbs (up to waist) immersed in hot water. The temperature ideally 40 degrees but here we can maintain the water temperature as per the bearing capacity of the child. For instance, if the child is comfortable at 39 degrees, then you can maintain the water temperature at 39 degrees for 30 minutes, twice a day. This is a very critical part of the entire treatment protocol.

Here you must take care of a minor detail. The patients of Thalassemia or blood transfusion patients become prone to developing a fever or flu as part of a side-effect of the transfusion itself. As explained in the previous chapter, this is known as delayed hemolytic reaction. This means the side effect of the transfusion persists even after two to three weeks of the procedure and the patient, as a result, develops flu or flu-like symptoms.

When the patient experiences fever, then instead of lower limb hot water immersion technique, just restrict the treatment to his lower leg region. Here the water temperature needs to be maintained at 42 degrees. For young children 42 degrees of temperature might a bit too much to bear, so they can immerse their lower legs in or around 40 to 42 degrees temperature. The primary focus should be the comfort level of the child and this procedure can be followed two to three times a day, every time for about 30 mins, till the child gets relief from fever.

## Lower Leg Hot Water Immersion to overcome fever

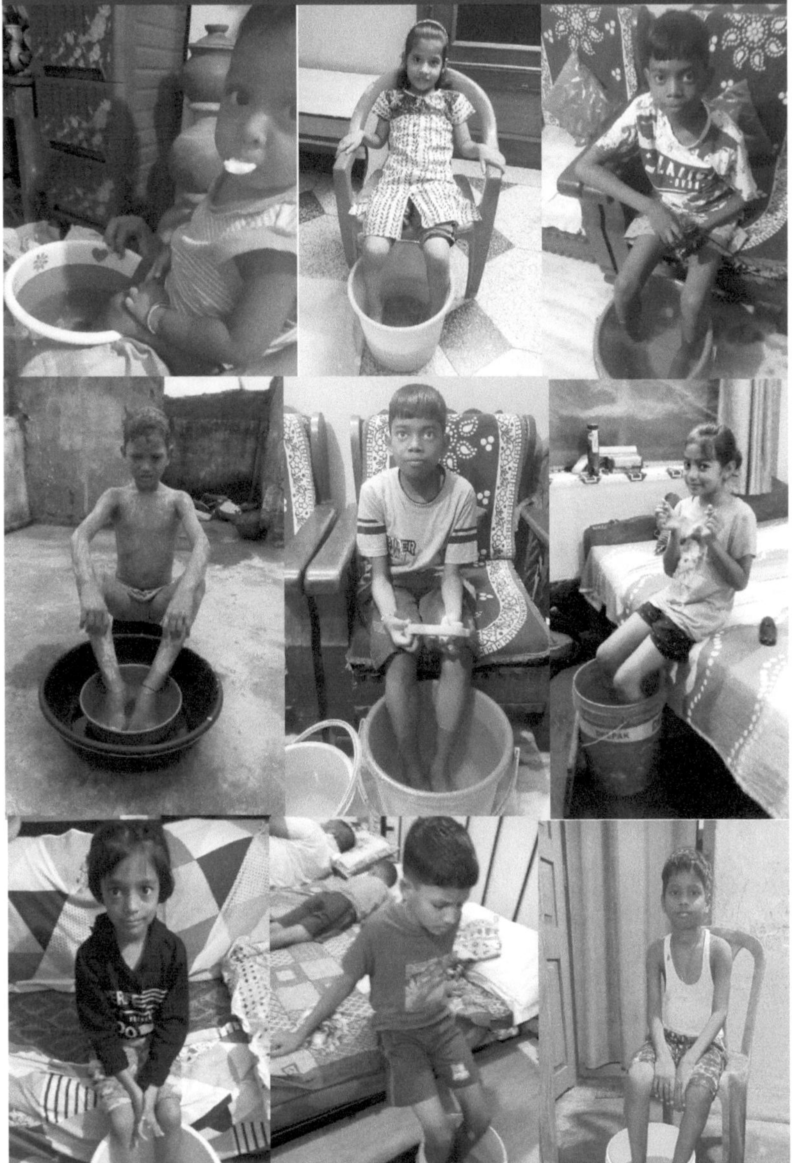

On regular days when the child does not experience flu or flu-like symptoms we use Lower Limb Hot Water Immersion Therapy. However, on days when the child is unwell with fever, we will shift the treatment from Lower Limb to Lower Leg and continue the treatment as Lower Leg Hot Water Therapy.

## Step 6 – Hobbies

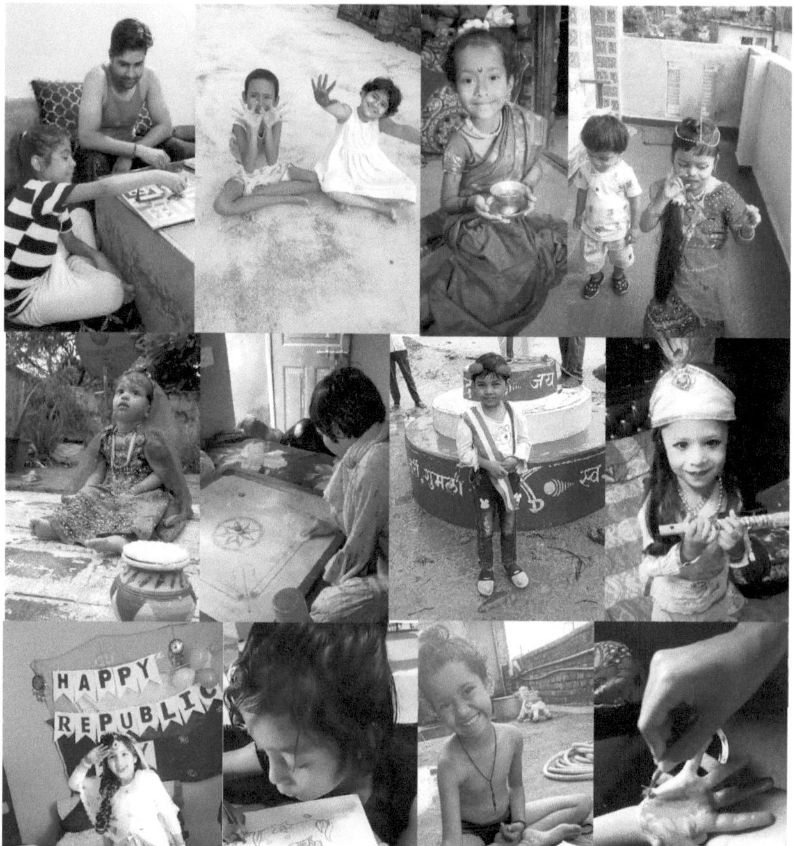

This is the final step and the most neglected dimension of our lives. You can observe any household with a child who keeps unwell, where the family is told that the child can never be cured of the disease, and there is an associated financial burden due to prolonged treatments and hospital bills. Such homes are sad with a dull and heavy atmosphere.

It is important to understand that the atmosphere of our homes holds an important role in the health and recovery of patients. It has been scientifically proven that when the patient pursues a hobby that interests him, or if he works towards a specific purpose in his life which is positive in nature, then his chances of recovery increase manifold.

**Relationship of Having Hobbies and a Purpose in Life With Mortality, Activities of Daily Living, and Instrumental Activities of Daily Living Among Community-Dwelling Elderly Adults**

Chances of cancer is Double,
Chances of stroke increases by 80%,
Chances of Diabetes increases by 20%,
Chances of Heart disease increases by 40%,
among the people without having hobbies in comparison to people with hobbies

*Kimiko Tomioka, Norio Kurumatani, and Hiroshi Hosoi*
*Nara Prefectural Health Research Center, Nara Medical University, Kashihara, Nara, Japan*
*Received June 5, 2015; accepted September 23, 2015; released online March 5, 2016*

In this chapter we are laying focus on the various conditions that help in the improvement of the health condition of the patient. Of these factors, the most neglected factor is the patient pursuing a hobby which brings joy and fulfilment to his life. This helps him fulfil some purpose in life.

We have incorporated this as an essential step in the healing process of all of our patients by leading them to pursue any positive goal or purpose in life. It can be anything they feel most akin to, like collection of things like stamps, or beautiful stones, playing board games like skipping a rope, dancing to a new song every day, etc.

We can help inculcate a sense of competition, or a series of activities leading to the fulfillment of a goal in the patient. We notice when the child starts developing interest in the same, or when we create an environment of fun and joy for the patient to pursue and work towards completing a goal, it has been observed the speed of recovery in the child increases. In addition, we have also observed a significant reduction in the obvious symptoms of anemia and blood transfusion in the body of the child diagnosed with Thalassemia. Pursuing hobbies is an integral part of the Living Water Therapy. So now we can understand living water is not just the water we drink when we feel thirsty. Every living thing is made of water, for instance the fruits and vegetables and even the human body. When we are in our mother's womb, we are 96% made of water. At birth, we are 80% made of water and now as adults we all comprise 70% water, and the water content of the body often reduces to 50%.

We have closely observed all our patients who undergo blood transfusion. When we incorporate all the six steps of the Living Water Therapy as part of their treatment protocol, we are able to observe a visible improvement in the health condition of those children within the first 24 hours itself. We can find evidence of significant improvement in terms of the child's energy levels, the quality of their sleep, his level of alertness and various such aspects within the first 24 to 48 hours of implementing the Living Water Therapy.

As a caretaker of the patient, when you are helping the patient towards adopting the Living Water Therapy, you need to keep a check on various factors with respect to anemia and its associated details. You need to be mindful of the different check points and the various triggers while undergoing living water therapy.

You would be required to be extremely alert and scrutinizing so as to identify which trigger point must be considered as an alarm when the blood transfusion becomes a more favorable choice. In other words, the triggers leading to blood transfusion become a lesser dangerous factor as compared to living with anemia itself.

So in order to gain a deeper perspective surrounding anemia, you first need to understand when a patient's body develops anemia over an extended period of time, the body develops a compensatory mechanism. Here the patient starts adjusting to lower hemoglobin which depends on the etiology, the speed of onset and chronicity of anemia.

**In sickle cell Anemia with holding RBC transfusion despite profound anemia, results in cessation of hemolysis and reconstitution of bone marrow erythropoiesis**

*Win N, Doughty H, Telfer P, Wild B, Pearson T. Hyperhaemolytic transfusion reaction in sickle cell disease. Transfusion. 2001;1:323-8.*
*Petz LD, Garratty G. Bystander immune hemolysis immune hemolytic anemias. 2nd ed. Philadelphia (PA): Churchill Livingstone; 2004, pp. 358– 64*

When the body suffers from anemia, it adopts certain compensatory changes.

These include the following:

- Increased cardiac output through increased stroke volume and myocardial contractility
- Variable contribution of increased heart-rate
- Decreased peripheral vascular resistance
- Decreased blood viscosity and rightward shift in oxy-hemoglobin
- Disassociation curb and subsequent increase in oxygen offloading to the tissues

As the anemic condition worsens in the body, it reflects the following changes:

- With hemoglobin levels at 6 to 7 gram per deciliter, the cardiac output increases steeply peaking at 180% of normal.
- With hemoglobin levels at 3 to 5 gram per deciliter, coronary blood flow shifts from endocardium to epicardium. This signals eminent danger in an otherwise healthy patient.

**In various studies, laboratory animals (dog and baboons), have tolerated a hemoglobin level as low as 3-5 gm/dl without major adverse effects.**

*Mangano DT, Hollenberg M, Fegert G, Meyer ML, London MJ, Tubau JF, Krupski WC. Perioperative myocardial ischemia in patients undergoing noncardiac surgery-I: Incidence and severity during the 4 day perioperative period. The Study of Perioperative Ischemia (SPI) Research Group. J Am Coll Cardiol. 1991 Mar 15;17(4):843-50.*

The optimal level of hemoglobin level is difficult to define in an anemic patient in a defined way due to a large number of factors differing with the compensatory mechanism.

| **The minimally acceptable Hb level for sustained tissue life was defined as approximately 3g/dl which corresponds to the critical delivery of oxygen that coincides with the metabolic shift from aerobic to anaerobic** |
| --- |
| *Spence RK and Mintz PD. Transfusion in Surgery, Trauma and Critical Care. In: Mintz PD, ed. Transfusion Therapy: Clinical Principles and Practice, 2nd ed. Bethesda, MD: AABB Press, 2005: 203– 41.*<br>*Pearlman ES, Ballas SK. When to transfuse blood in sickle cell disease? Lessons learned from Jehovah's* |

The minimally acceptable hemoglobin level for sustaining tissue life was defined in the 1930s by Carel and Lindburg as approximately 3 grams per deciliter. This corresponds to the critical delivery of oxygen that coincides with the metabolic shift from aerobic to anaerobic.

An analysis of the case report of a patient who refused blood transfusion due to religious reasons concluded that nearly all deaths of patients with hemoglobin levels less than five gram per deciliter happened.

| **In sickle cell disease RBC transfusion may do more harm than good** |
| --- |
| *Josephson CD, Su LL, Hillyer KL, Hillyer CD. Transfusion in the patient with sickle cell disease: a critical review of the literature and transfusion guidelines. Transf Med Rev. 2007;21:118–33.* |

The meta-analysis of clinical trials evaluating the impact of using restrictive process liberal transfusions trigger confirmed the initial finding of the TRICC trail that mortality rates were lower with the restrictive transfusion strategy among the younger, less acutely ill patients.

**Despite comparable baseline characteristics and severity of illness, patients who were transfused liberally suffered more in-hospital deaths (23.3% vs 18.7%), higher adjusted multiple organ dysfunction score (11.8 vs 10.7), and more complications [combined cardiac complications (21.0% vs 13.2%), myocardial infarctions (2.9% vs 0.7%), and pulmonary oedema (10.7% vs 5.3%)] during intensive care unit (ICU) stay.**

*Hebert PC, Wells G, Blajchman MA, et al. A multicenter, randomized, controlled clinical trial of transfusion requirements in critical care. Transfusion Requirements in Critical Care Investigators, Canadian Critical Care Trials Group. N Engl J Med 1999; 340: 409–17*

Among many adverse reactions around the transfusion one of the major adverse reaction is called TRALI (Transfusion Related Acute Lung Injury), which is often known to cause irreparable damage or even death of the patient. That is why blood transfusion is sometime known as more dangerous than the anemia.

**Impact of renal insufficiency, anaemia, and transfusions on in-hospital mortality was examined in 596 456 patients. All three components (anaemia, renal insufficiency, and transfusion) were independently associated with mortality, and transfusion reinforced the detrimental effects of the other two.**

*176 Kao DP, Kreso E, Fonarow GC, Krantz MJ. Characteristics and outcomes among heart failure patients with anemia and renal insufficiency with and without blood transfusions (public discharge data from California 2000–2006). Am J Cardiol 2011; 107: 69–73*

Based on the available evidences, we should not panic as long as our hemoglobin is above 4 gram per deciliter specially if the patient is asymptomatic.

**RBCs should not be used for the treatment of asymptomatic compensated chronic anemia or merely to improve a person's sense of wellbeing.**

*A compendium of transfusion practice guidelines American Red Cross First Edition; 2010.*

Conclusively, I must say Thalassemia is not a genetic disorder. It does not exist in the child's body because of the genes of the parents. Rather, it exists due to the factors which are totally preventable. The factors determining the increased chances of being diagnosed with anemia, or getting trapped in a vicious circle of being a Thalassemia patient, as discussed, can be summarized as follows:

Vaccination - the greatest of all the causes of Thalassemia.

Fever- It is important to note any child when suffering with fever as a rule experiences a temporary decrease in the hemoglobin levels. When the fever subsides, hemoglobin levels of the child's body also return back to normal, as discussed. However, if one interferes with the fever with antipyretic drugs and the child is also administered with antibiotic medications, or for any other reason, the child is given any kind of drugs and medicines; it can also result in the patient's body being induced with anemia.

Animal Protein – If a young child is given animal proteins on a regular basis, for instance, any dairy product like milk, curd, ghee, buttermilk, cheese, butter, cow milk and its derivative products, or eggs, fish and meat, for some children it results in triggering an auto-immune reaction. This may result in the destruction of Red Blood Cells in the child's body leading to an anemic situation.

For most of the children, despite having all these conditions, their body continues to be on a recovery mode and gradually reverses itself to a healthy condition. However, if we interfere with the body's system by adopting the blood transfusion procedure, then blood transfusion itself causes a great amount of damage. This leads to the weakening of the child's body's own ability to manufacture Red Blood Cells. A temporary anemic situation may sometimes be converted into a permanent disease called Thalassemia.

CHAPTER -3

# Cancer Cure

What is Cancer? You can redefine cancer as anemia, especially in case of end-stage cancer. You can see a direct correlation between the reduction in hemoglobin and an increase in the tendency of cancer.

Let us now understand the connection and correlation between anemia and cancer. Here it goes!

Anemia causes tumor hypoxia, which often leads to Angiogenesis. As a result of Angiogenesis the tumor aggressiveness increases. This condition is regarded as cancer.

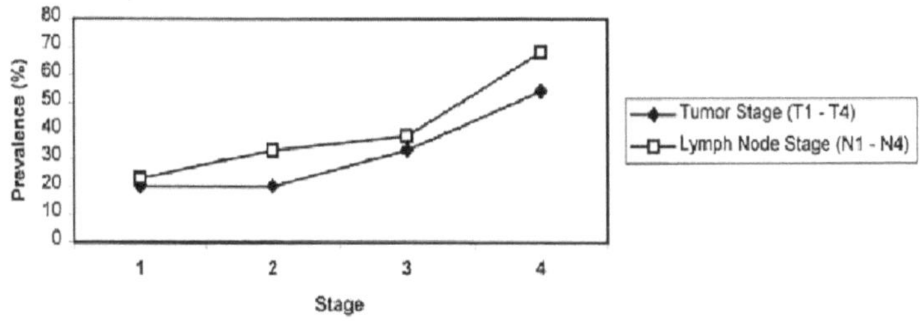


**Prevalence of anemia by tumor and lymph node stages in patients with head and neck cancers. Anemia prevalence increases with disease severity, rising 3-fold from the earliest to the most advanced tumor stage and slightly less to the most advanced lymph node stage.**

*Dubray B, Mosseri V, Brunin F, et al. Anemia is associated with lower local-regional control and survival after radiationtherapy for head and neck cancer: a prospective study. Radiology. 1996;201:553–558.*

As you can see in the table given below, whether it is the lung cancer, breast cancer, ovarian cancer or the cancer of the uterine cervix, leukemia, bone cancer, and even the Non-Hodgkin's Lymphoma and pancreatic cancer. On an average 90% of the patients, towards the end-stage of the cancer also suffer from anemia.

| |
|---|
| **84% of patients with lung cancer had anemia.**<br>**82% of patients with breast cancer had anemia.**<br>**85% of patients with ovarian cancer had anemia.**<br>**93% of pancreatic cancer had anemia** |
| *Tchekmedyian NS. Anemia in cancer patients: significance, epidemiology, and current therapy. Oncology (Huntingt). 2002;16(suppl 10):17–24.* |

| |
|---|
| **93% of patients with lymphoma had anemia.**<br>**97% of pediatric patients with leukemia had anemia.**<br>**78% of the bone cancer patient were found anemic.** |
| *Michon J. Incidence of anemia in pediatric cancer patients in Europe: results of a large, international survey. Med PediatrOncol. 2002;39:448–450.* |

The correlation between anemia and cancer can also be concluded from the graph given below which shows the evidence of anemia by disease prevalence in patients with renal cancer.

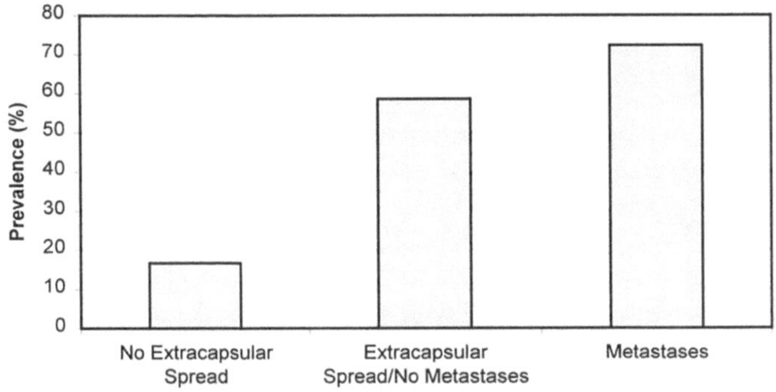


**Prevalence of anemia by disease-severity in patients with renal cancer! Anemia prevalence increases about 4-fold with extracapsular spread and grows further with metastasis.**

*vonKnorring J, Selroos O, Scheinin TM. Haematologic findings in patients with renal carcinoma.Scand J UrolNephrol. 1981;15:279–283.*

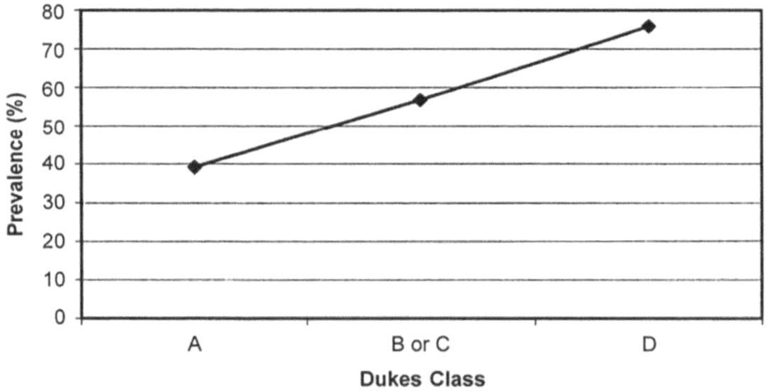


**Prevalence of anemia in hospitalized patients with colon cancer varies with disease severity: 40% of patients with Dukes stage A tumors had anemia, compared with nearly 80% of patients with stage D tumors.**

*Cappell MS, Goldberg ES. The relationship between the clinical presentation and spread of colon cancer in 315 consecutive patients: a significant trend of earlier cancer detection from 1982 through 1988 at a university hospital. J ClinGastroenterol. 1992;14:227–235.*

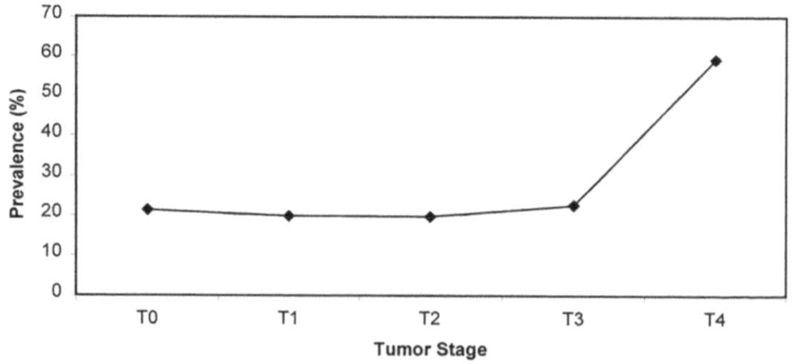


**Prevalence of anemia in patients with prostate cancer appears relatively stable at about 20% in stages T0–T3; progression to stage T4 is associated with a 3-fold increase in prevalence.**

*Dunphy EP, Petersen IA, Cox RS, Bagshaw MA. The influence of initial hemoglobin and blood pressure levels on results of radiation therapy for carcinoma of the prostate. Int J RadiatOncolBiol Phys. 1989;16:1173–1178.*

We can interpret this direct relation between anemia and end-stage cancer as a ray of hope. This means logically if we could remove anemia or increase the hemoglobin level in the body of the cancer patient, chances of the survival and of improving the quality of life of the patient should also proportionately improve as is suggested from various clinical studies.

**The cross-sectional study reported an association between anemia and both functional and well-being scores.**

*Cella D. The Functional Assessment of Cancer TherapyAnemia (FACT-An) Scale: a new tool for the assessment of outcomes in cancer anemia and fatigue. SeminHematol. 1997;34(suppl 2):13–19.*

This suggests that if you wish to cure a cancer patient, then you must focus on the most important aspect of removing all those factors that result in an anemic condition, reduce the hemoglobin levels, or result in the destruction of RBC in the body. These factors have been discussed in great detail in the first chapter.

If we take a look at these essential factors once again, then the most important one that needs to be guarded against is avoiding all kinds of animal food. Secondly, one must keep a look-out for avoiding all kinds of drugs.

As you would know that the treatment prescribed for cancer in modern medicine is chemotherapy and radiation. However, in reality both chemotherapy and radiation lead to anemia and destruction of RBCs in the body. In addition, both lead to the reduction of hemoglobin levels in the body. One can argue that chemotherapy as well as radiation procedures result in a dangerously uncontrolled reduction in hemoglobin in the system.

**Prevalence of anemia in patients with cervical cancer was 67% before radiation therapy and 82% afterwards.**

*Harrison LB, Shasha D, White C, Ramdeen B. Radiotherapy-associated anemia: the scope of the problem. Oncologist. 2000;5(suppl 2):1–7.*

In any respect, neither chemotherapy nor radiation is given to a patient to cure, control, or even prevent the cancer growth in the body. It is rather a mode to help the cancer spread throughout the system. I have been communicating about the adverse effects of chemotherapy and radiation to all my patients over the last several years. As you can see the references are provided in the boxes. All the references given below conclude only one thing that chemotherapy is not a cure for cancer, but promotes cancer growth in the patient's body.

**Blood Health:**
Chemotherapy decreases red blood cells (anemia)[1]
Chemotherapy decreases white blood cells (leukopenia)[2]
Chemotherapy decreases blood platelets [3]

**Bone Health:**
Chemotherapy causes bone death (osteonecrosis) [4]
Chemotherapy causes loss of bone mineral density (osteopor-osis) [ 5-6]

**Brain Health:**
Chemotherapy is toxic to the brain (neurotoxic) [7]
Chemotherapy causes long-lasting impairment of concentration, forgetfulness and slower thinking; termed "chemobrain [8-9]
Chemotherapy causes altered consciousness [10]
Chemotherapy causes degeneration of white matter in the brain(leukoencephalopathy)[10]
Chemotherapy causes damage(neuropathy) [10]
Chemotherapy causes seizures [10]
Chemotherapy causes paralysis[10]
Chemotherapy causes stroke (cerebral infarction)[10]

**Digestive Health:**
Chemotherapy causes diarrhoea[18]
Chemotherapy causes painful inflammation and ulceration in the digestive tract (intestinal mucositis) [23]
Chemotherapy causes "significant intestinal damage in both jejunum and colon" [19]

**Exercise:**
Chemotherapy reduces grip strength [20]
Chemotherapy causes muscle dysfunction and a loss of overall strength [21]

**Eye Health:**
Chemotherapy causes severe vision loss and altered colorvision [22]

Chemotherapy causes complete blindness [23]

**Hair Health:**
Chemotherapy causes hair-loss [30]

**Healing:**
Chemotherapy impairs wound healing [31]

**Hearing:**
Chemotherapy causes "severe to profound hearing loss" [32]
Chemotherapy causes chronic ringing of the ears (tinnitus) [32]

**Heart Health:**
Chemotherapy damages the heart [33]
Chemotherapy causes heart disease [34]
Chemotherapy causes heart failure [35]
Chemotherapy causes heart attacks (myocardial infarction) [36]

**Immune System:**
Chemotherapy causes long-term immune system damage [37-38]
Chemotherapy exacerbates existing hepatitis C infections [39]
Chemotherapy reactivates hepatitis B virus [40]
Chemotherapy impairs anti-tumor immune response [41]

**Kidney Health:**
Chemotherapy causes kidney failure [42]

**Liver Health:**
Chemotherapy causes liver injury [43]

**Lung Health:**
Chemotherapy causes lung disease [44]

Mental Health:
Chemotherapy "decreased emotional and social function and increased distress" [11]
Chemotherapy causes depression [12]
Chemotherapy causes anxiety [13]

**Oral Health:**
Chemotherapy causes severe dental caries [14]
Chemotherapy causes dry mouth (xerostomia), ulcers and mouth sores [45]

Chemotherapy causes oral candida (fungal) infection [15]
Chemotherapy causes painful inflammation and ulceration in the mouth (oral mucositis) [16]
Chemotherapy causes "a diverse spectrum of oral changes that generally are attributed to im-munosuppression and bleeding tendencies" [17]

**Pain:**
Chemotherapy causes neuropathic pain; burning or coldness, "pins and needles" sensations, numbness and itching [46]
Chemotherapy pain remains one-year after treatment [47]

**Quality of Life:**
Chemotherapy causes diffculty swallowing (dysphagia) [48]
Chemotherapy causes nausea and vomiting (emesis) [49-50]
Chemotherapy causes altered taste sensation [51]
Chemotherapy causes migraine headaches.[52]

**Sexual Health:**
Chemotherapy causes infertility and premature ovarian failure [24-25] in up to 66% of women [26]
Chemotherapy causes absence of menstrual period (amenorrhea) [27]
Chemotherapy causes menopausal symptoms [27]
Chemotherapy damages sperm and testicular tissue [28-29]
Chemotherapy reduces reproductive organ weight; sperm count and sperm motility [28]

***For references go to www.biswaroop.com/onequestion***

If among the readers of this book, we also have cancer patients, it is advised to stop chemotherapy and radiation immediately no matter at what stage of treatment you are in. Do not even consider taking an appointment for the next session.

Now let us understand how can we cure Cancer completely? For this, one needs to go back to the previous chapter and adopt the Living Water Therapy. The method which helped to get rid of the dependency on blood transfusion will also help in preventing, controlling even reversing cancer.

I would like to conclude this section of the book with a strong recommendation for all kinds of cancer patients to follow the 'Living Water Therapy'. It must be followed for a minimum of six to nine months consistently to get optimum results.

# SECTION -II

**On the occasion of the birth anniversary of Shaheed Chandra Shekhar Azad and Lokmanya Bal Gangadhar Tilak (i.e on 23rd July 2022), we opened entry for the Thalassemia patients to participate in our virtual "Living Water Therapy" program conducted by Dr. Namita (MBBS, MD) We closed the registration with the participation count reaching 150 patients.**

**In the pages ahead we included the testimonials of the patients who could follow the Living Water Therapy at least 50% or more. There testimonials are based on the 1st 40 days of observation, after the patients adopted the Living Water Therapy.**

**For video testimonials of the patients, go to www.coronakaal.tv/thalassemia**

# Success Stories

## 1

Baidyanath Hota age 4.5 years, son of Rushikesh Hota( runs his own business) and mother Manaswini Satapathy ( a homemaker), resides in Bissamcuttack, Odisha. Baidyanath Hota was diagnosed with thalassemia for the first time at the age of 6 months. Just before the diagnosis he had jaundiced skin and was vomiting a lot. The doctor advised to go for blood test and that was the first time thalassemia was diagnosed. Since then he has been taking treatment at AIIMS, Bhubaneswar.

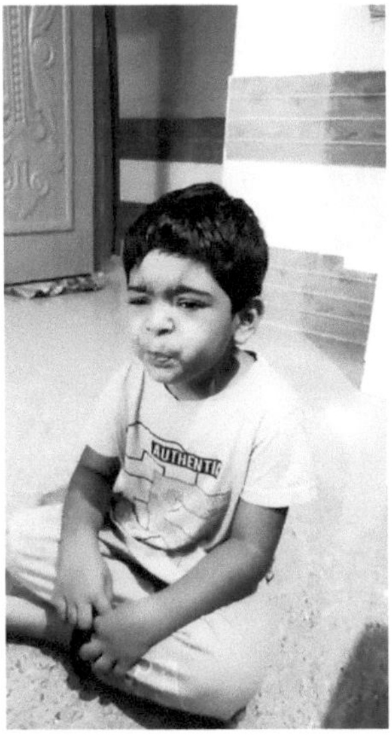

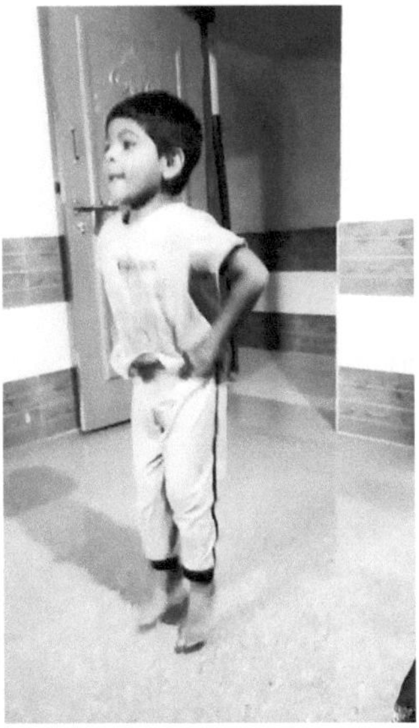

Following were Baidyanath's parameters before starting Living Water Therapy:

**Frequency of transfusion:** once in 20 to 25 days

**Lowest Hemoglobin/ Hb ever recorded:** 5.2

**Medication taken:** Folic Acid, Deferasirox, Shelcal, Zincovit CL

**Physical Symptoms /Discomforts:** Anxious/ restless mind, low intake of food, yellow eyes and skin, fatigue

They came into our contact on 5-Aug-22 and started Living Water Therapy.

The present status after starting the therapy

**Frequency of Transfusion:** Nil

**Medications:** Nil

**Physical Symptoms/ Discomforts:** Nil

*Father Rusikesh Hota's relief and joy knows no bounds since the day they started the Living Water Therapy. He sums up in just 2 words about his views on Living Water Therapy & Dr Biswaroop Roy Chowdhury, "Godfather of my child".*

## 2

Akshita Chawla age 11 years, daughter of Tarun Chawla (runs his own business) and mother Shalu Chawla (a homemaker), resides in New delhi, Delhi. Akshita Chawla was diagnosed with thalassemia for the first time at the age of 6 months. Just before the diagnosis she had fever. Doctor advised to go for blood test and that was the first time thalassemia was diagnosed. Since then she has been taking treatment at Sir Ganga Ram Hospital - Delhi.

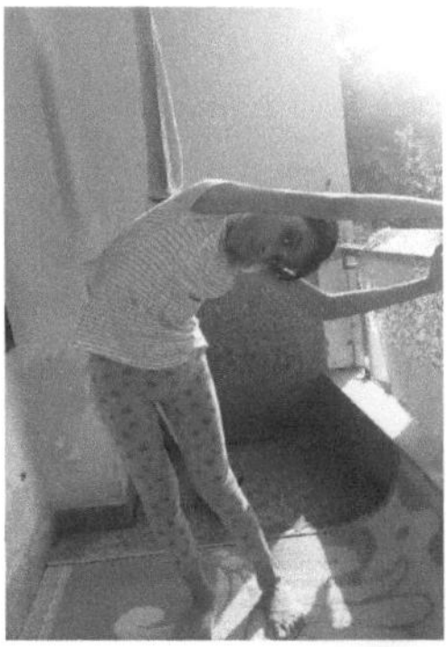

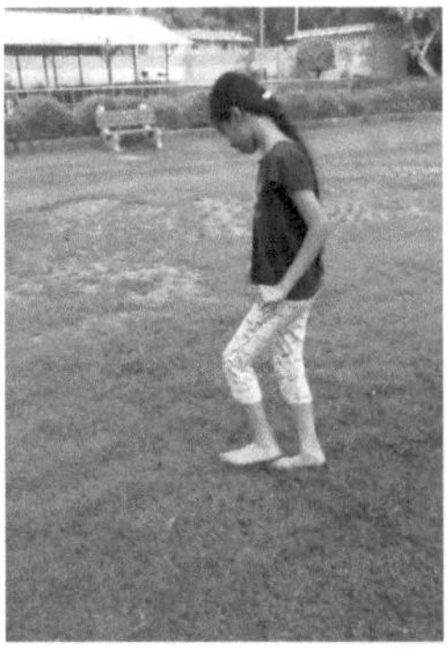

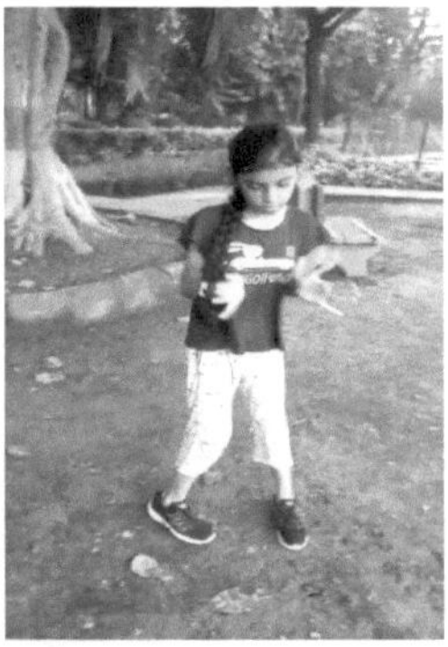

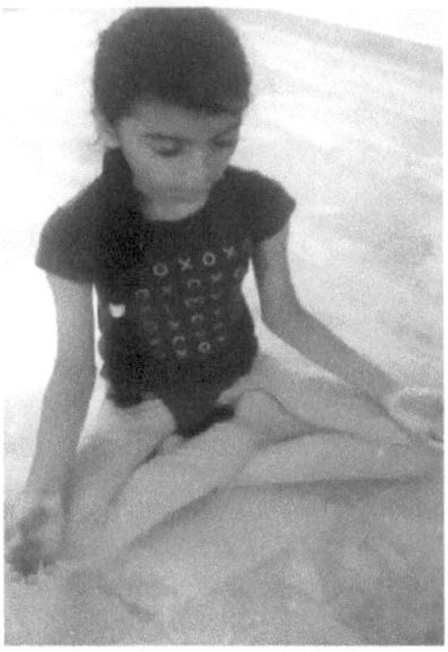

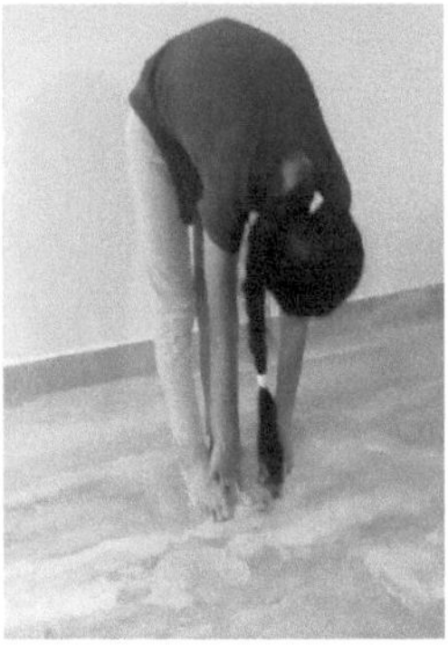

Following were Akshita's parameters before starting Living Water Therapy:

**Frequency of transfusion:** once in 23 days

**Lowest Hemoglobin/ Hb ever recorded:** 4.5

**Medication taken:** Kelfer, Defrijet

Physical Symptoms /Discomforts: recurring Stomach aches

They came into our contact on 2 Aug 22 and started Living Water Therapy.

The present status after starting the therapy

**Frequency of Transfusion:** Nil

**Medications:** Nil

**Physical Symptoms/ Discomforts:** Nil

*Akshita's mother Shalu conceived with 3rd child when told by doctors that the born marrow transplant from the umbilical cord and stem cell therapy is possible. So she saved the stem cells. But the procedure failed. She was running from one hospital to the other for her daughter's transplant. The doctors assured her for transplant asap. But her family opposed it. Looking for cure the helpless mother came across a video on 'Khoon ka Rishta, the Living Water Therapy' as cure for thalassemia. She immediately enrolled for this program. Since then there have been no visits to any hospital or any transfusions. She is happy that her daughter is healed.*

# 3

Prisha Khanna age 8 years, daughter of Pradeep Khanna (works in ophthalmic industry) and mother Ruchi khanna ( a teacher), resides in Uttam Nagar, Delhi. Prisha Khanna was diagnosed with thalassemia for the first time at the age of 1 year. Just before the diagnosis she had recurring fever every month and weakness. Doctor advised to go for blood test and that was the first time thalassemia was diagnosed. Since then she has been taking treatment at AIIMS Delhi.

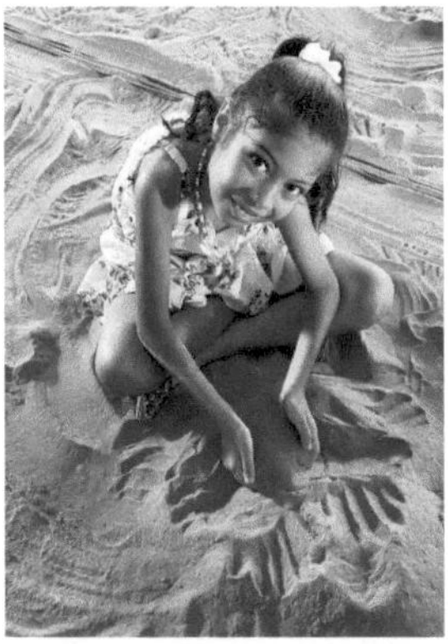

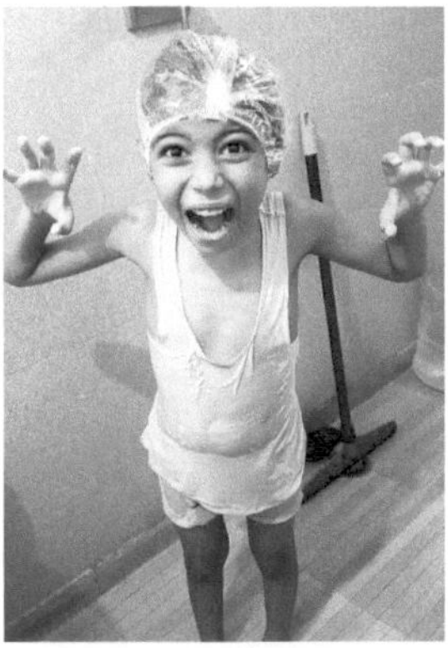

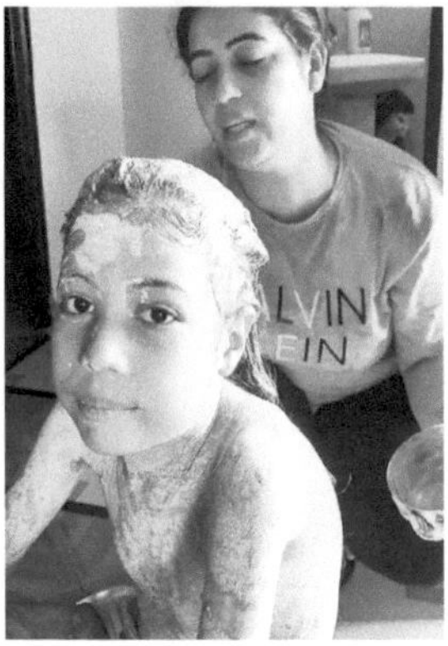

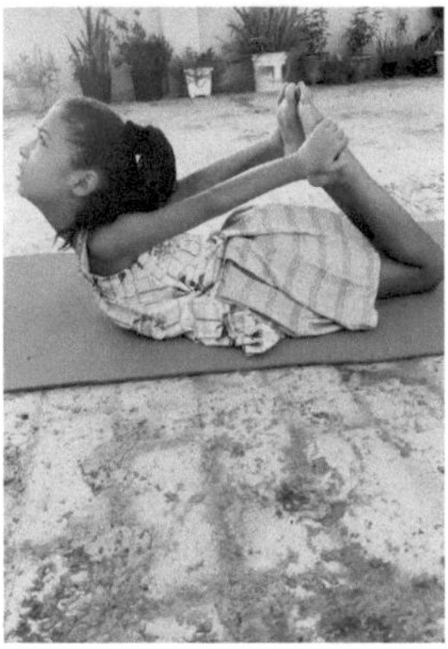

Following were Prisha Khanna parameters before starting Living Water Therapy:

Frequency of transfusion: once a month

**Lowest Hemoglobin/ Hb ever recorded:** 5.5

**Medication taken:** Defrijet, shelcal, folitas

**Physical Symptoms /Discomforts:** Weakness

They came into our contact on 23-Jul-22 and started Living Water Therapy.

The present status after starting the therapy

**Frequency of Transfusion:** Nil

**Medications:** Nil

**Physical Symptoms/ Discomforts:** weakness occassionally

*Father Mr Pradeep Khanna was shocked to know that Prisha is a suspected thalassemic patient when on 26 August 2022, he rechecked Prisha's diagnostic reports upon insistence by Dr. Namita Gupta our team member who is supervising Living water therapy Program. He feels cheated and robbed by "Red Mafia" at the cost of his daughter's health life.*

# 4

Aerika age 5 years, daughter of Ravi kumar (a Software engineer at HCL Noida) and mother Rinku Rani (a homemaker), resides in Patiala, Punjab. Aerika was diagnosed with thalassemia for the first time at the age of 7 month. Just before the diagnosis she had fever. Doctor advised to go for blood test and that was the first time thalassemia was diagnosed. Since then she has been taking treatment at Rajendra Hospital Patiala.

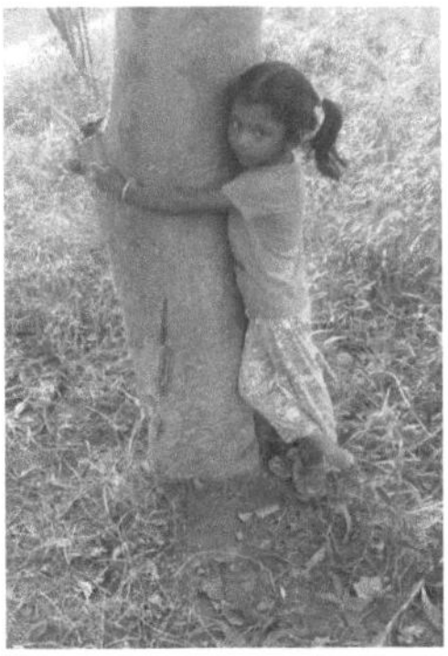

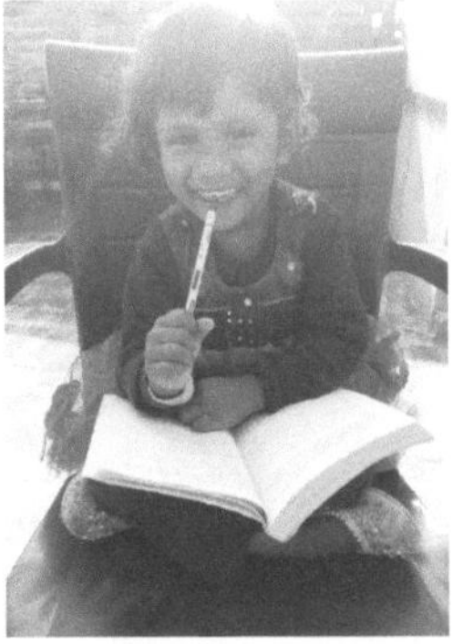

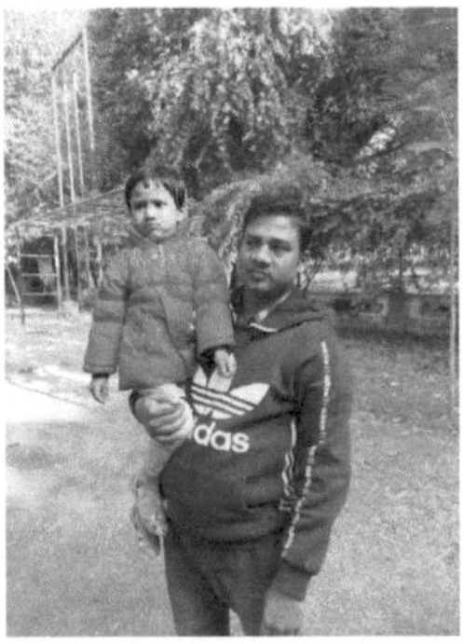

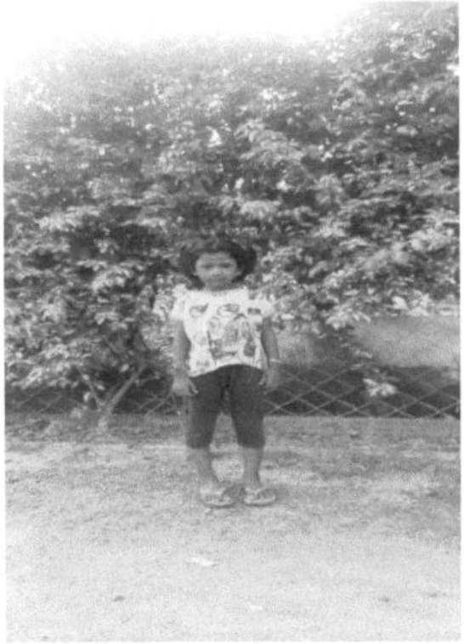

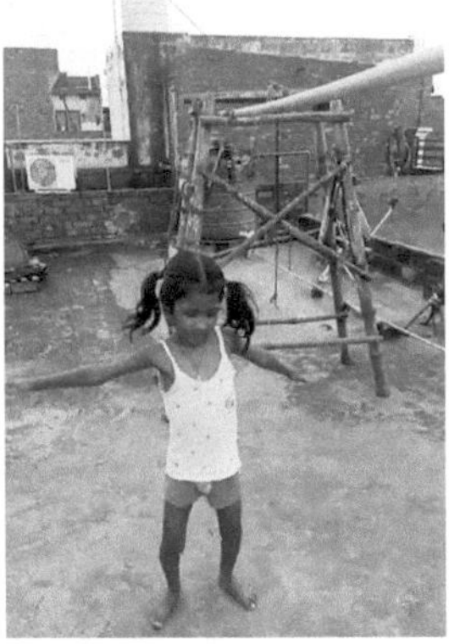

Following were Aerika parameters before starting Living Water Therapy:

**Frequency of transfusion:** once in 22 days

**Lowest Hemoglobin/ Hb ever recorded:** 8.5

**Medication taken:** Chlorofill, Tab to reduce iron overload

**Physical Symptoms /Discomforts:** Fever and tiredness

They came into our contact on 21-Jul-22 and started Living Water Therapy.

The present status after starting the therapy

**Frequency of Transfusion:** Nil

**Medications:** Nil

**Physical Symptoms/ Discomforts:** Nil

*Aerika's father is thankful to god that his child was saved just in time as they were about to go for bone marrow transplant costing around INR 20-25 lakhs. The procedure for surgery had already started just then Living Water Therapy started. He cancelled the surgery immediately and enrolled for the Living water Therapy. Since that day there is no turning around. His child is completely cured. He now wishes to leave his corporate job and want to go back to his native place in Gaya UP in the lap of nature and want to treat other thalassemic children who still are struggling to stay alive!*

# 5

Samarjit Mahato age 5 years, son of Kumud Kishor Mahato (runs his own business) and mother Santoshi Mahanta (employed with Odisha State Police), resides in Mahipani, Odisha. Samarjit Mahato was diagnosed with thalassemia for the first time at the age of 8 months. Just before the diagnosis he had weakness, vomiting. Doctor advised to go for blood test and that was the first time thalassemia was diagnosed. Since then he has been taking treatment at CMC Vellore.

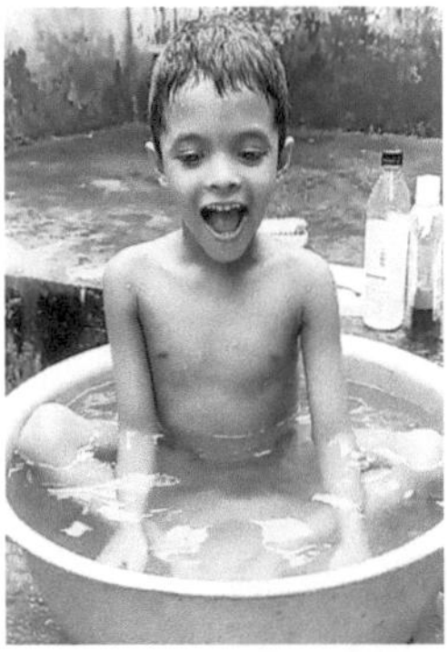

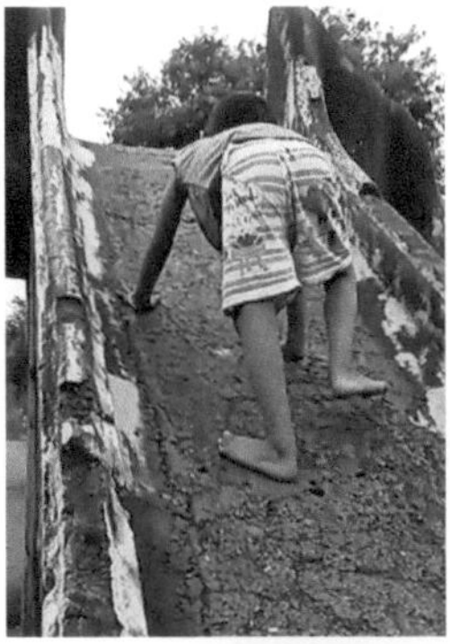

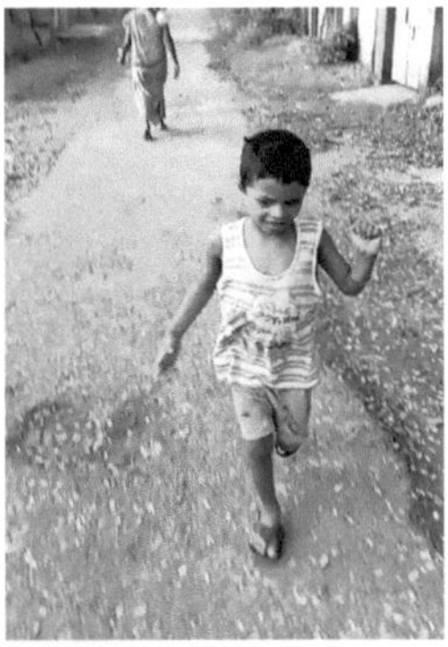

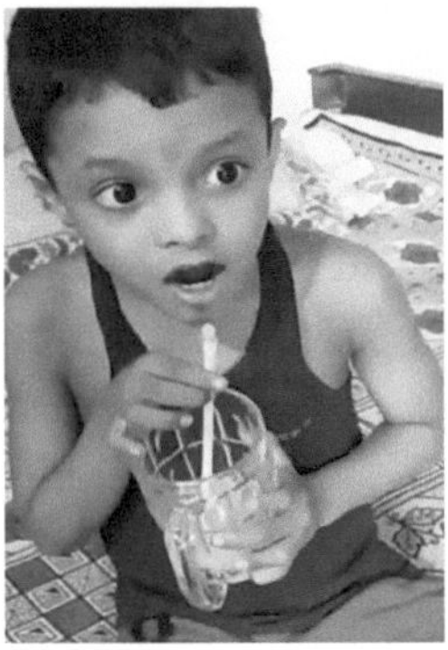

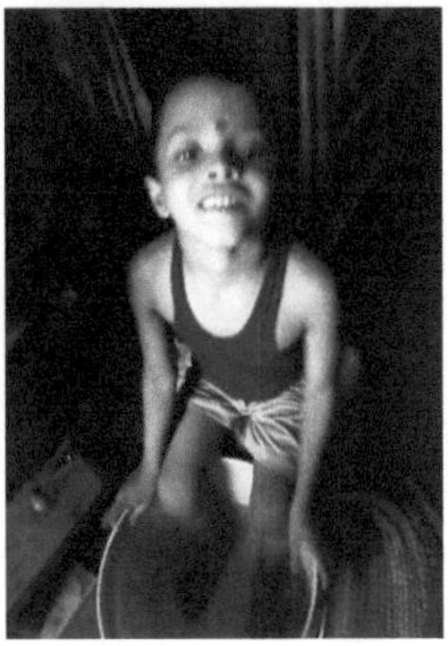

Following were Samarjit Mahato parameters before starting Living Water Therapy:

**Frequency of transfusion:** once a month

**Lowest Hemoglobin/ Hb ever recorded:** 5

**Medication taken:** Defrijet 500, folic acid

Physical Symptoms /Discomforts: Weakness, cold n cough

They came into our contact on 16-Aug-22 and started Living Water Therapy.

The present status after starting the therapy

**Frequency of Transfusion:** Nil

**Medications:** Nil

**Physical Symptoms/ Discomforts:**

*Mother comments, "It is a very good program and a ray of hope for all the children as well as parents who are in mentally shocked situation due to monthly blood transfusion and ruined health in future.*

# 6

Maheshwari Vilin Dhotre age 5 years, daughter of Vilin Devidasrao Dhotre(an office Peon, Shri Shivaji College of Arts, Comm. & Science, Akola.) and mother Prajakta Vilin Dhotre ( a homemaker), resides in Akola, Maharashtra. Maheshwari Vilin Dhotre was diagnosed with thalassemia for the first time at the age of 4 months. Just before the diagnosis, they observed that her weight was not increasing, she was getting lazy and was not taking mothers milk properly. Her skin color was getting more and more pale yellowish and skin was not as shiny as other children at her age. Doctor advised to go for blood test and that was the first time thalassemia was diagnosed. Since then she has been taking treatment at City Central Hospital, Bhagde Complex Akola.

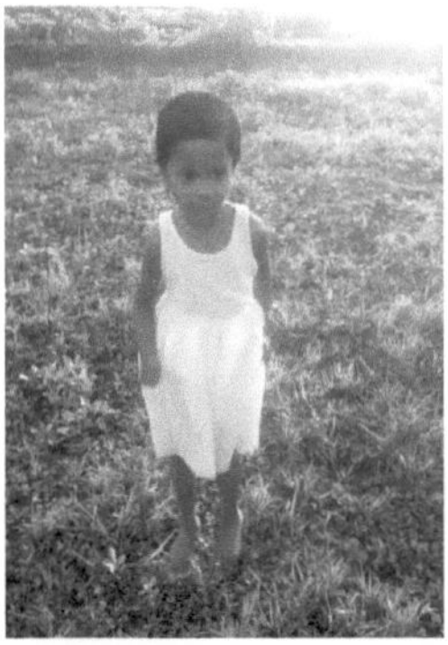

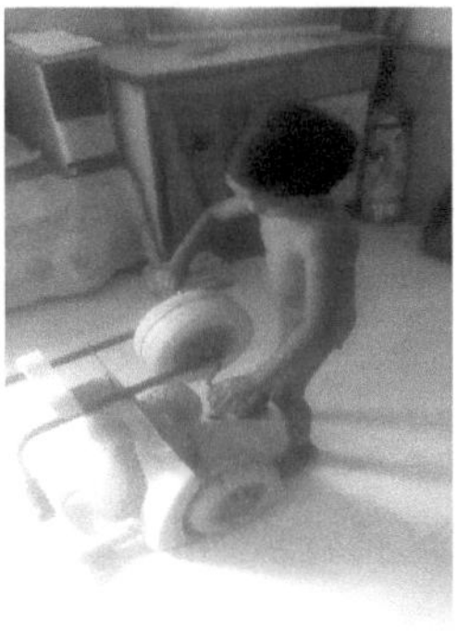

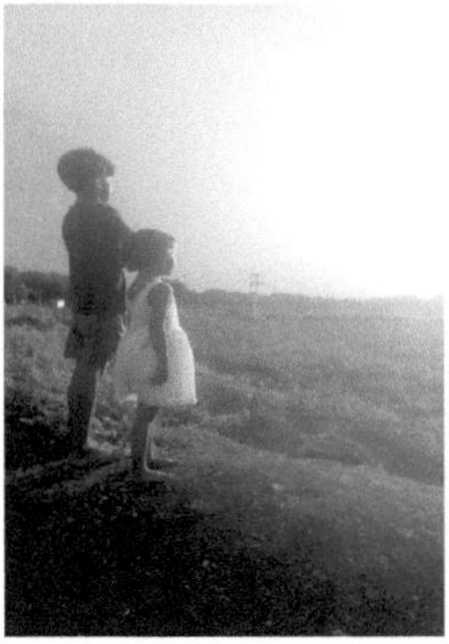

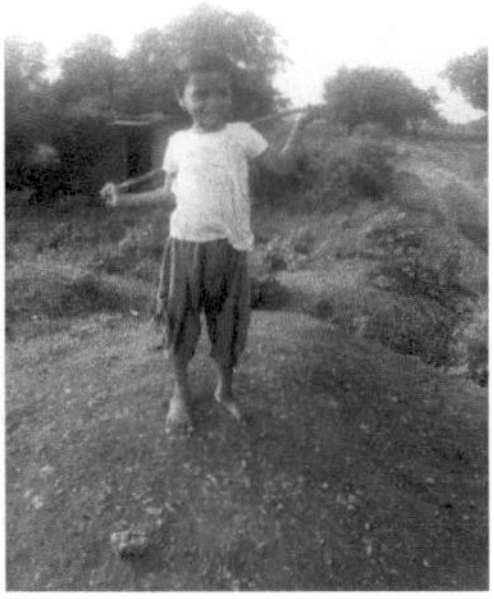

Following were Maheshwari 's parameters before starting Living Water Therapy:

**Frequency of transfusion:** once in 20-21 days

**Lowest Hemoglobin/ Hb ever recorded:** 6.2

**Medication taken:** Tab Defferosirox, Folic acid

**Physical Symptoms /Discomforts:** Loss of appetite, dullness, irritation, skin turning more and more pale yellow or whitish

They came into our contact 24-Jul-2022 and started Living Water Therapy.

The present status after starting the therapy

**Frequency of Transfusion:** Nil

**Medications:** Half tab. Defferosirox

**Physical Symptoms/ Discomforts:** Nil

*Father Vilin Devidasrao Dhotre shares, 'This is the best platform of humanity and giving a real help for everyone without money. This programme is saving life of lots of patients, extending the time & quality of life. For my family this program has given a new hope for our happiness. If anybody (parents of thalassemic patients) thinks that all the ways are closed then let me tell you, God can come in any form! For us its Dr BRC and his team. Trust and follow his advice and you will definitely get results.*

# 7

Abish Anjum age 9 years, son of Md. Abu Taleb (runs his own business) and mother Aleya Biswas (a homemaker), resides in Lalgola, West Bengal. Abish Anjum was diagnosed with thalassemia for the first time at the age of 2.5 Years. He used to cry all the time, so the parents took him to a doctor. The doctor advised to go for blood test and that was the first time thalassemia was diagnosed. Since then he has been taking treatment at Tata Medical Center .

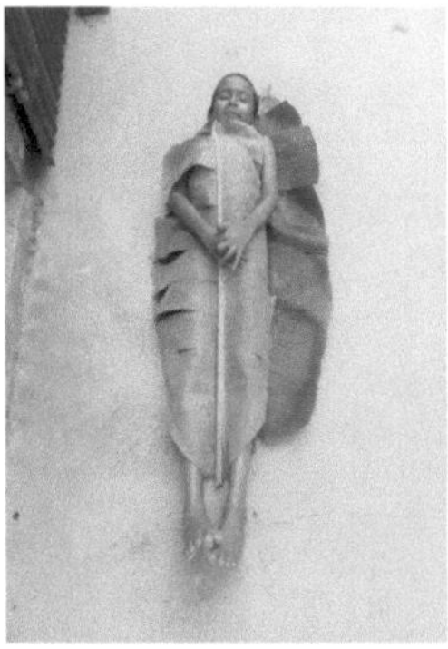
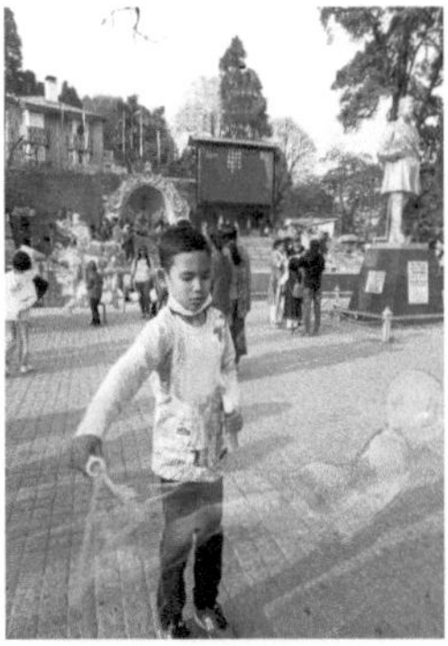
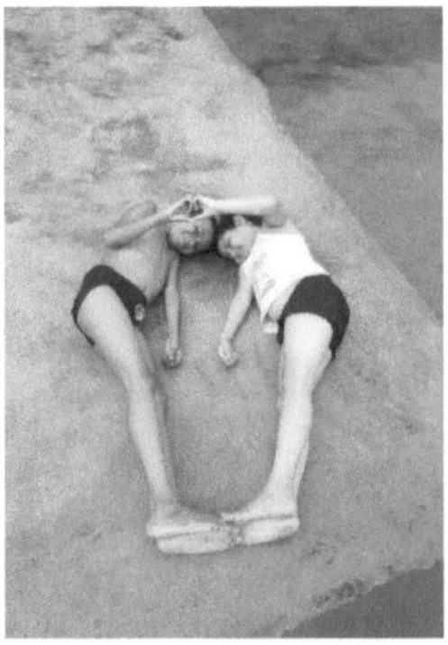
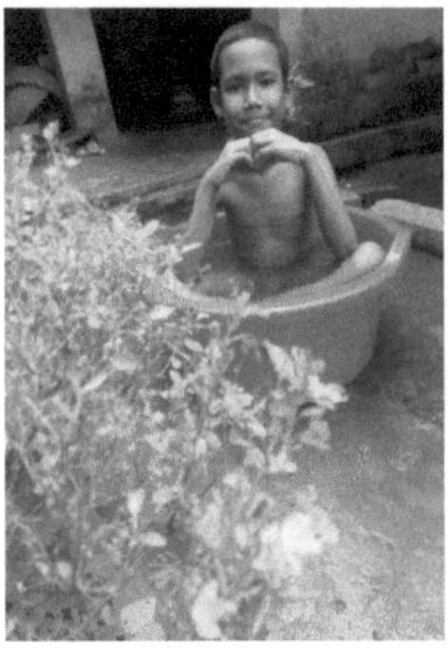
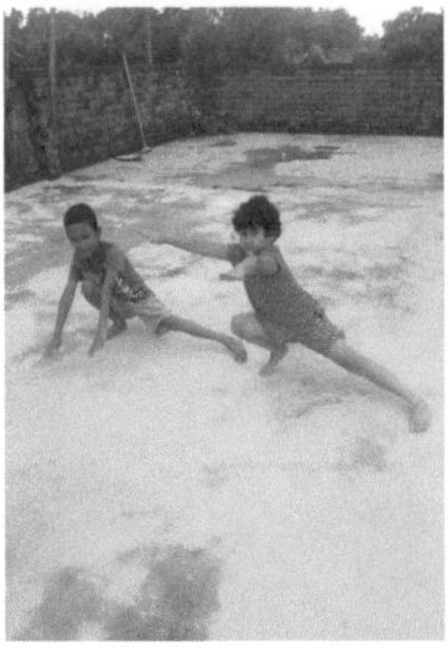
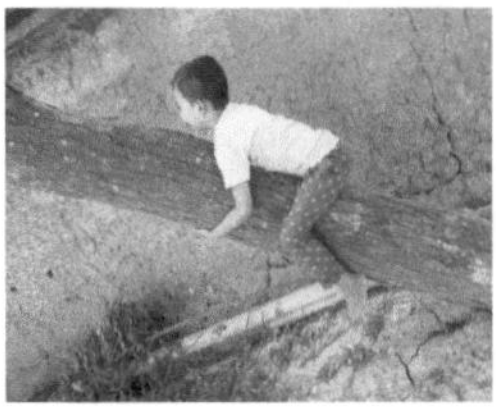

Following were Abish's parameters before starting Living Water Therapy:

**Lowest Hemoglobin/ Hb ever recorded:** 5.8

**Medication taken:** Hydra 500, Folvite

**Physical Symptoms /Discomforts:** Nil

They came into our contact on 10-Aug-22 and started Living Water Therapy.

The present status after starting the therapy

**Medications:** Nil

**Physical Symptoms/ Discomforts:** Nil

*Abhish's mother recalls the immense pain that child endured while doing tests before bone marrow transplant. It was heart wrenching for parents to see their child braving pain & suffering like this.*

*Running from pillar to post in search of cure for their child they finally found respite with 'Living Water Therapy'*

# 8

Hetaksh Zanzrukiya age 7 years, son of Manish (self smployed) and mother Nimisha (a homemaker), resides in Vadodara, Gujarat. Hetaksh Zanzrukiya was diagnosed with thalassemia for the first time at the age of 3 months. Observing his yellow skin, the parents decided to visit a doctor. The Doctor advised to go for blood test and that was the first time thalassemia was diagnosed. Since then he has been taking treatment at SSG Hospital.

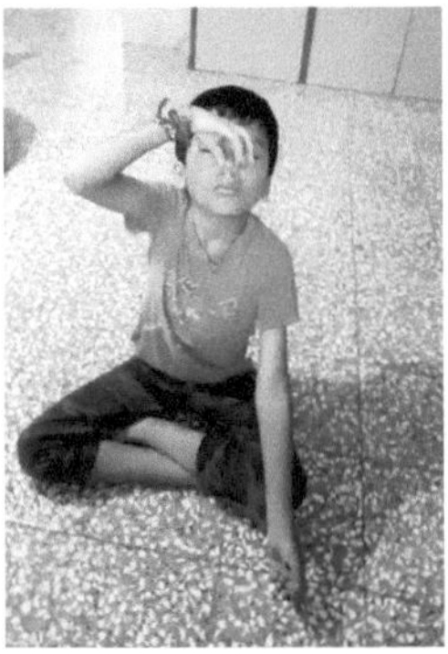

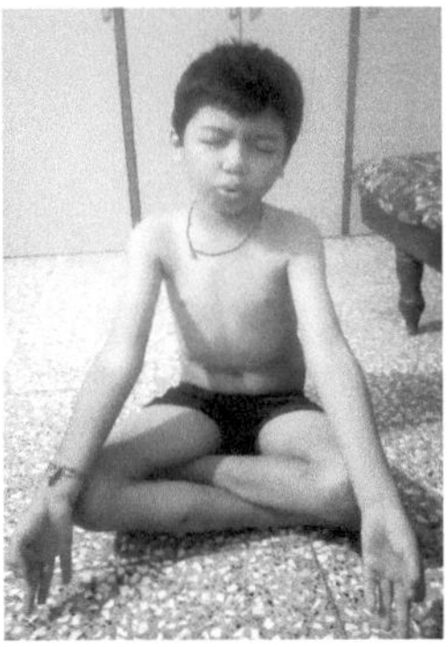

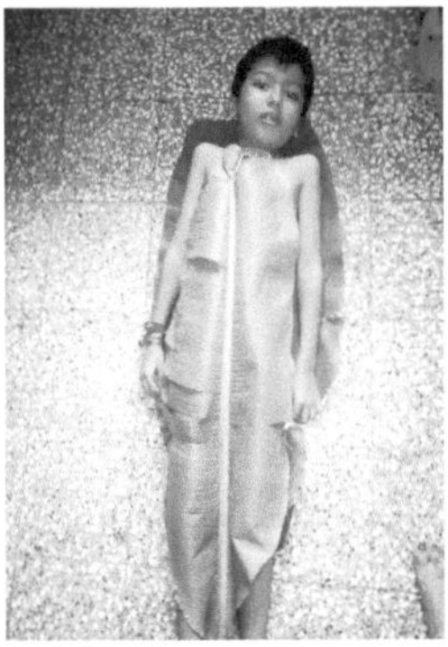

Following were Hetaksh's parameters before starting Living Water Therapy:

Frequency of transfusion: once in 21 days

**Lowest Hemoglobin/ Hb ever recorded:** 4.5

**Medication taken:** Desirox 500 mg

**Physical Symptoms /Discomforts:** Weakness, yellow skin

They came into our contact on 30 Jul 22 and started Living Water Therapy.

The present status after starting the therapy

**Frequency of Transfusion:** Nil

**Medications:** Nil

**Physical Symptoms/ Discomforts:** Nil

*Mother comments, "Hetaksh stringently follows the diet plan i.e. drinking coconut water, green and red juices, fruits, vegetables and plays and exercises a lot as advised. Whatever weakness he was feeling earlier is all gone now."*

# 9

Dibyansi Sahoo age 1 year 9 month, daughter of Prem Ranjan Sahoo ( engaged in a private job.) and mother Khirojtanaya Sahoo ( a homemaker), resides in Cuttack, Odisha. Dibyansi Sahoo was diagnosed with thalassemia for the first time at the age of 10 months. Just before the diagnosis she had fever, cold and cough. Doctor advised to go for blood test and that was the first time thalassemia was diagnosed. Since then she has been taking treatment at Kauvary Hospital Trichy.

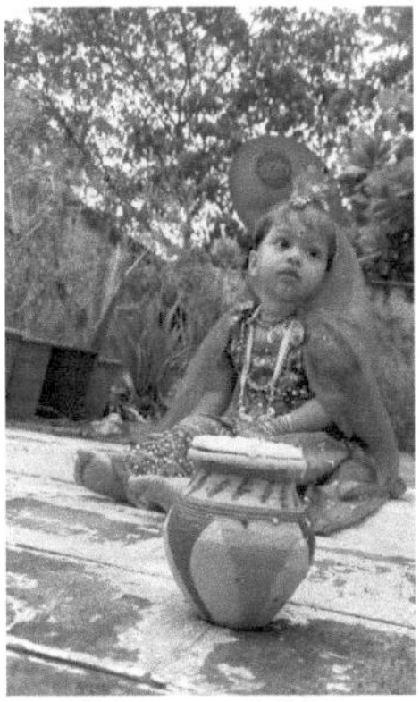
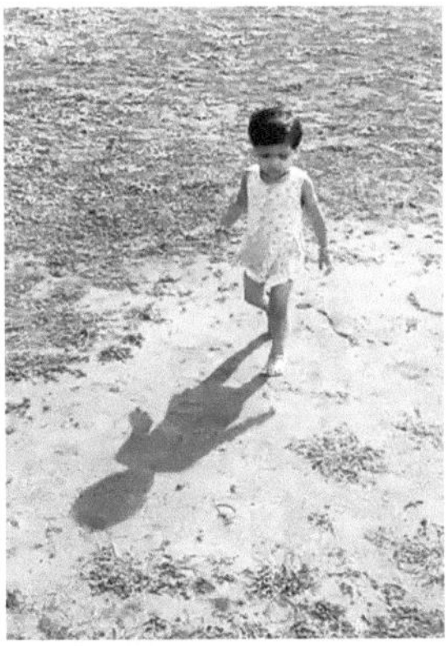
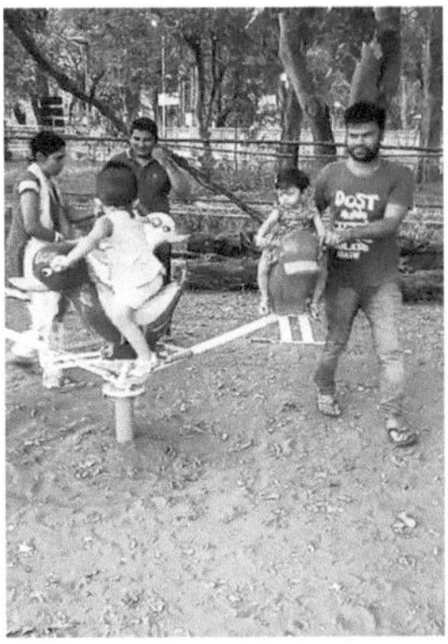
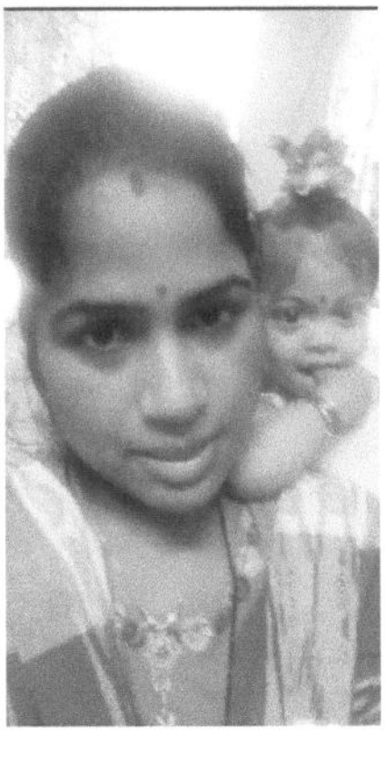
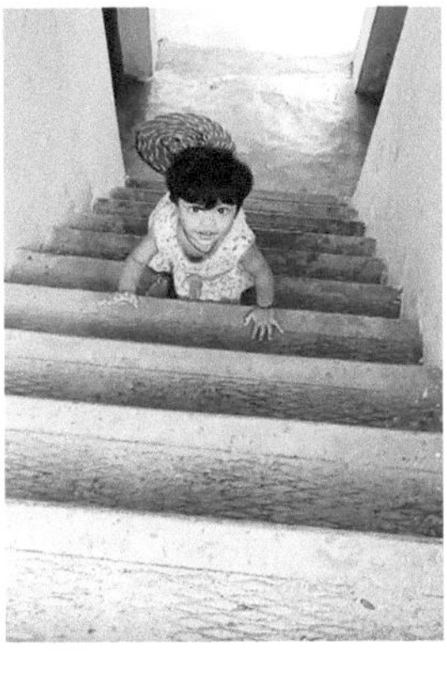
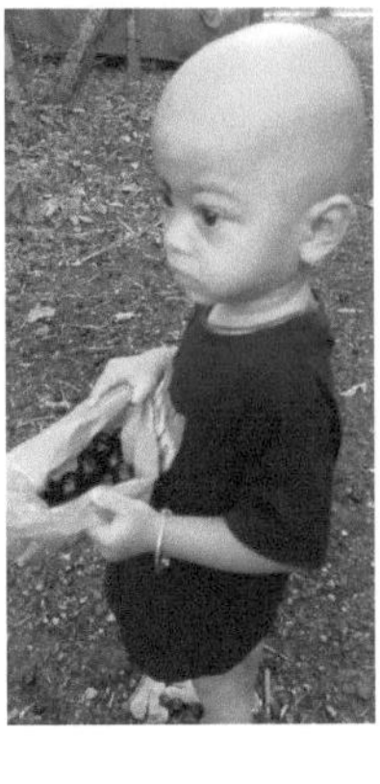

Following were Dibyansi's parameters before starting Living Water Therapy:

**Frequency of transfusion:** once in 4 weeks

**Lowest Hemoglobin/ Hb ever recorded:** 3

**Medication taken:** Syr Zincovit, Syr Shelcal, Tab Folvite

**Physical Symptoms /Discomforts:** Vomitting

They came into our contact on 25-Jul-22 and started Living Water Therapy.

The present status after starting the therapy

**Frequency of Transfusion:** Nil

**Medications:** Nil

**Physical Symptoms/ Discomforts:** had loose motions, fever, cold but recovered in one day

# 10

Anaya khan age 8 years, daughter of Akbar khan(an Ola cab driver) and mother Rabiya Begam ( a homemaker), resides in Mandideep, Bhopal, Madhya Pradesh. Anaya khan was diagnosed with thalassemia for the first time at the age of 18months. Just before the diagnosis she had physical weakness. Doctor advised to go for blood test and that was the first time thalassemia was diagnosed. Since then she has been taking treatment at Yashoda Hematology Clinic, Pune.

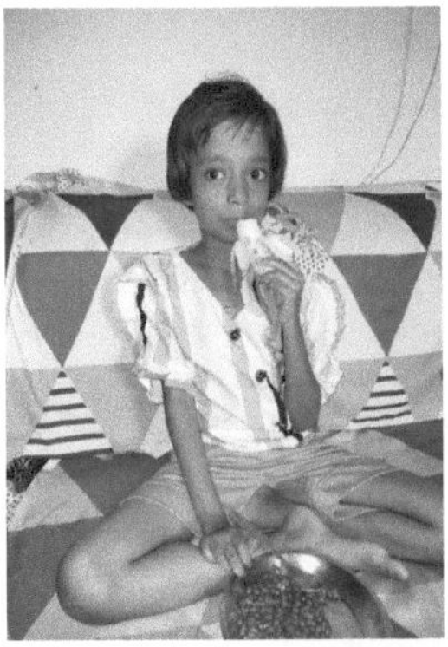
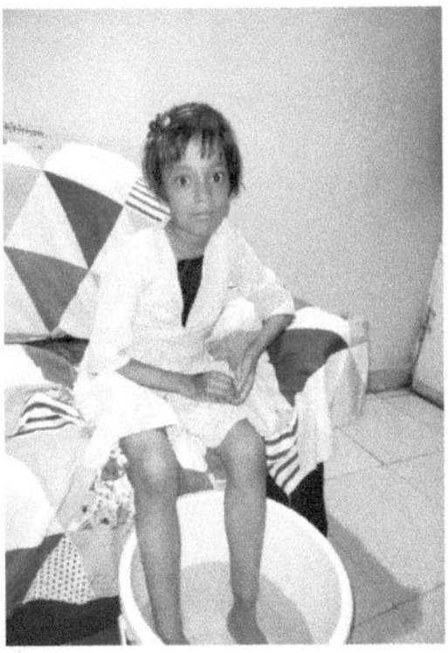
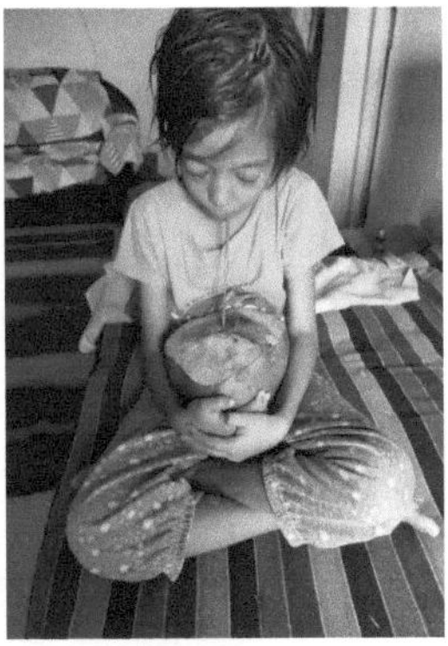
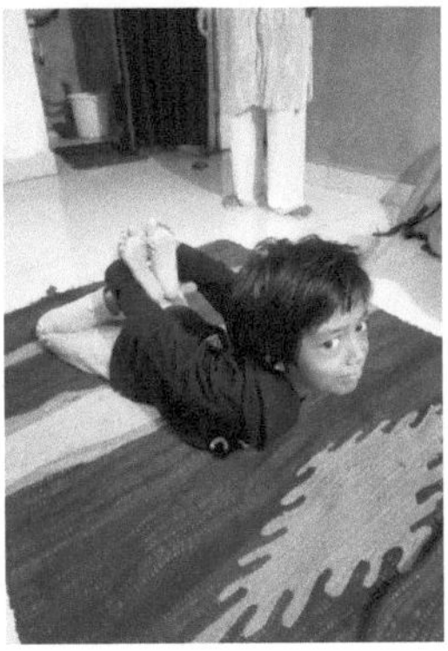
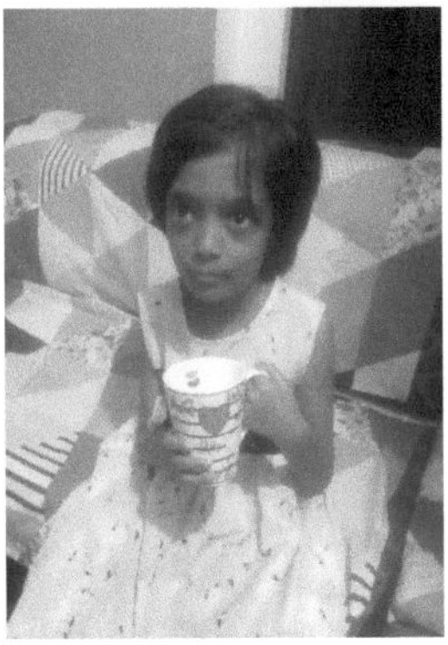

Following were Anaya khan parameters before starting Living Water Therapy:

**Frequency of transfusion:** once in 6 months

**Lowest Hemoglobin/ Hb ever recorded:** 3.5

**Medication taken:** Loprin, T-sapsure , T Glutamine, hydroxyurea, C2B plus, T numaxin, T Wysolone, T thalidomide

**Physical Symptoms /Discomforts:** Fever and Physical weakness

They came into our contact on 27 Jul 22 and started Living Water Therapy.

The present status after starting the therapy

**Frequency of Transfusion:** Nil

**Medications:** Nil

**Physical Symptoms/ Discomforts:** Nil

*Father's comments, "The simple and easy way to cure Thalassemia by Dr BRC has not only given new life to my child but also to the entire family. The whole family was suffering a lot seeing the child's painful life and no hope for future. But now we see a ray of hope. Thanks to Dr BRC.*

# 11

Mubashshira age 11 years, daughter of Mohammad Shakeel Ahmad (self Employed) and mother Hena Khatoon (a homemaker), resides in Begusarai, Bihar. Mubashshira was diagnosed with thalassemia for the first time at the age of 03 years. Just before the diagnosis she had jaundice. Doctor advised to go for blood test and that was the first time thalassemia was diagnosed. Since then she has been taking treatment at AIIMS Patna.

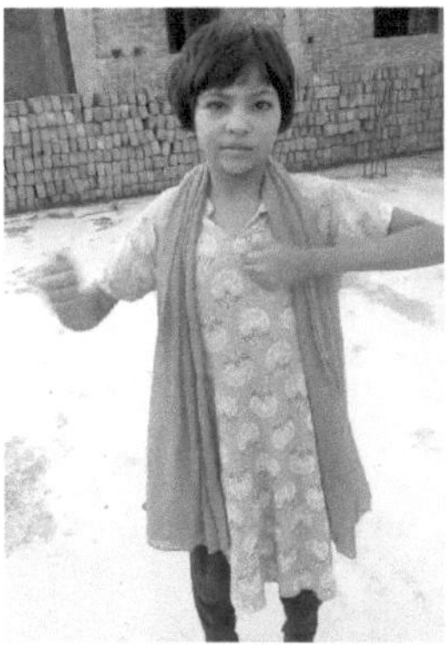
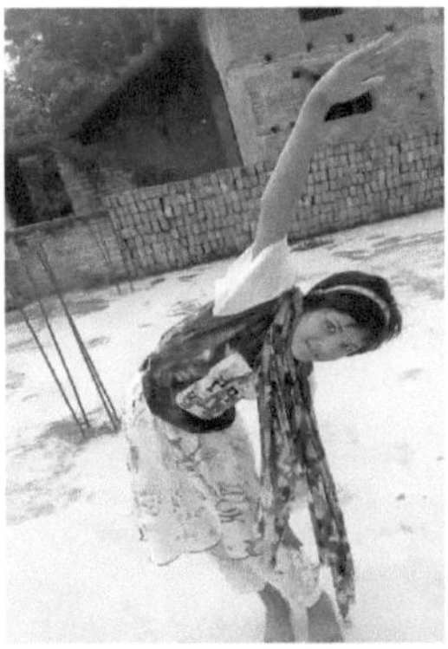
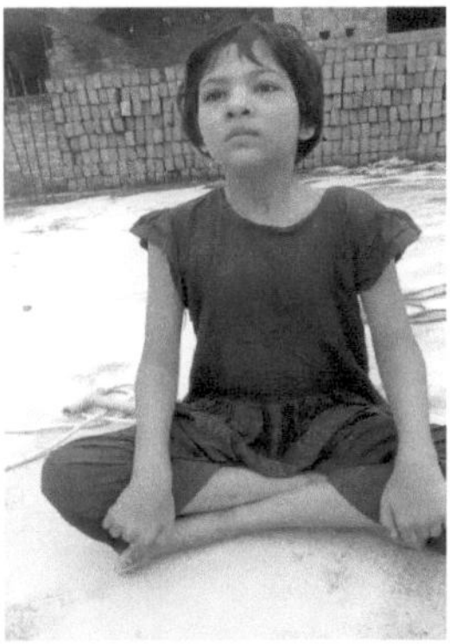
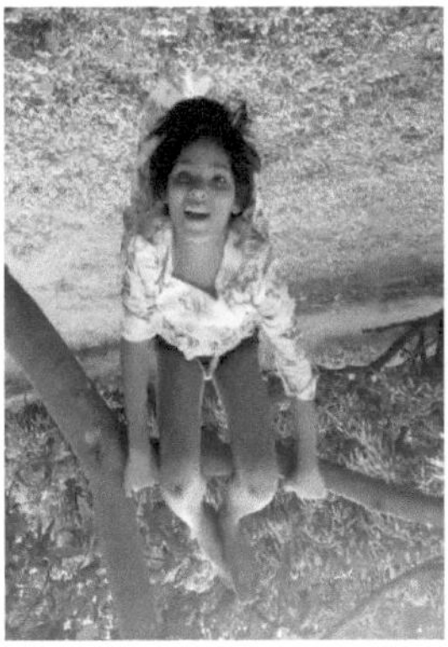
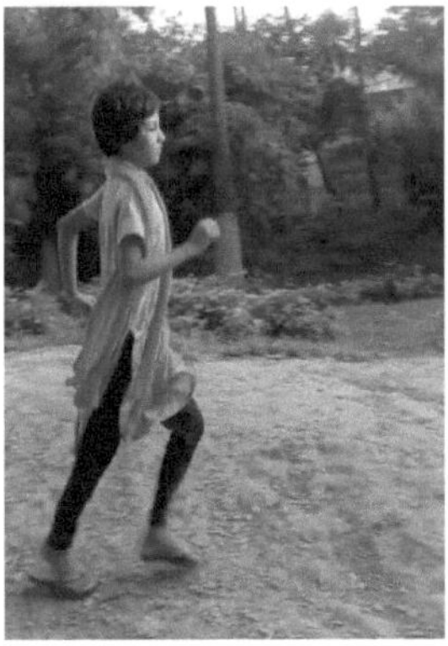

Following were Mubashshira parameters before starting Living Water Therapy:

**Frequency of transfusion:** once a month.

**Lowest Hemoglobin/ Hb ever recorded:** 4

**Medication taken:** Hydrosar 750 mg, ME12, desirox 500, Shelcal 20 mg

Physical Symptoms /Discomforts: Headache, pain in hand and legs.

They came into our contact on 29-Jul-22 and started Living Water Therapy.

The present status after starting the therapy

**Frequency of Transfusion:** Nil

**Medications:** Nil

**Physical Symptoms/ Discomforts:** headache sometimes

*Mother remarks, "Within 15 days of following the Living Water therapy Hb level went up from 7.1 to 8.1. Results were more than what we expected. Heartfelt thanks to Dr BRC and Dr Namita.*

# 12

Sharik Almas age 8 years, son of Shakeel sheikh (runs his own business) and mother Shama khan ( a homemaker), resides in Sieoni, MP. Sharik Almas was diagnosed with thalassemia for the first time at the age of 9 month. Just before the diagnosis he had jaundiced skin. Doctor advised to go for blood test and that was the first time thalassemia was diagnosed. Since then he has been taking treatment at Shree Child Clinic Nagpur.

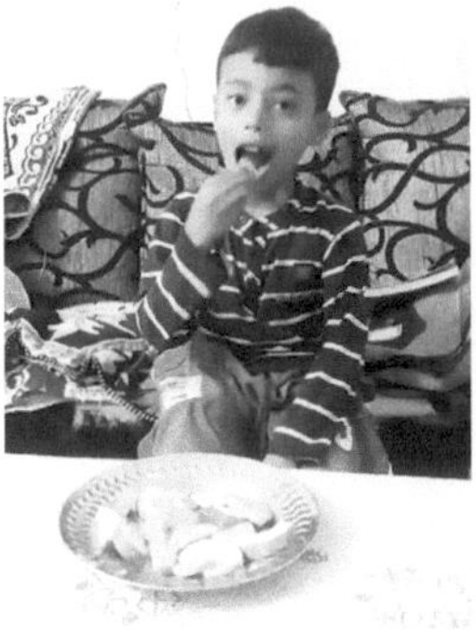
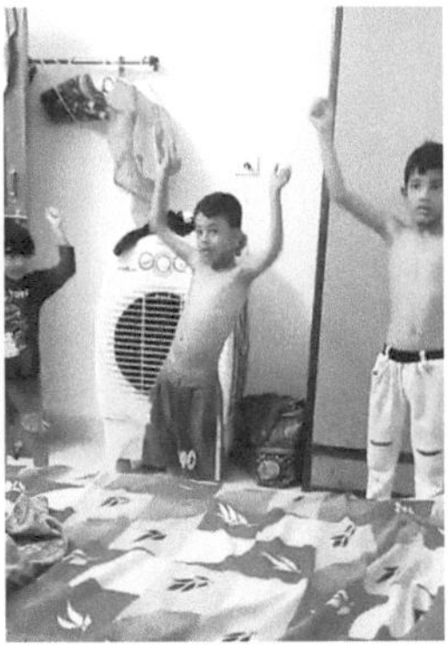
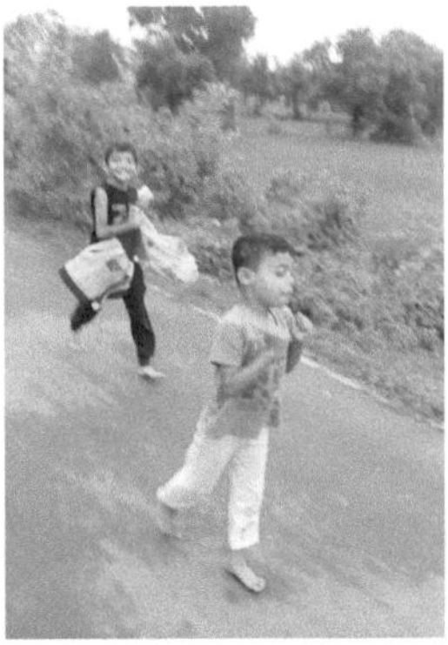

Following were Sharik Almas parameters before starting Living Water Therapy:

**Lowest Hemoglobin/ Hb ever recorded:** 5

**Medication taken:** Desirox, c2b, Ubiniche, Lasix, Glutaup

**Physical Symptoms /Discomforts:** refusing to eat food all the time

They came into our contact on 21-Jul-2022 and started Living Water Therapy.

The present status after starting the therapy

**Medications:** Nil

**Physical Symptoms/ Discomforts:** Nil

*Urging Dr BRC to continue the Living Water Therapy Program the father comments, "Dr BRC is an angel sent by God. I have just one request- please don't stop this Living Water Therapy program. This is last hope for Thalassemia patients. We still have to reach and cure lakhs of thalassemic patients."*

# 13

Dev Kashyap age 13 years, son of Kunjbihari Kashyap(a runs his own business) and mother Rama Kashyap ( a homemaker), resides in Bilaspur, Chhattisgarh. Dev Kashyap was diagnosed with thalassemia for the first time at the age of 10 and a half years diagnosed with Aplastic anemia. Just before the diagnosis he had blue patches on the body. Doctor advised to go for blood test and that was the first time thalassemia was diagnosed. Since then he has been taking treatment at Sanjivini CBCC USA cancer hospital Raipur Chhattisgarh.

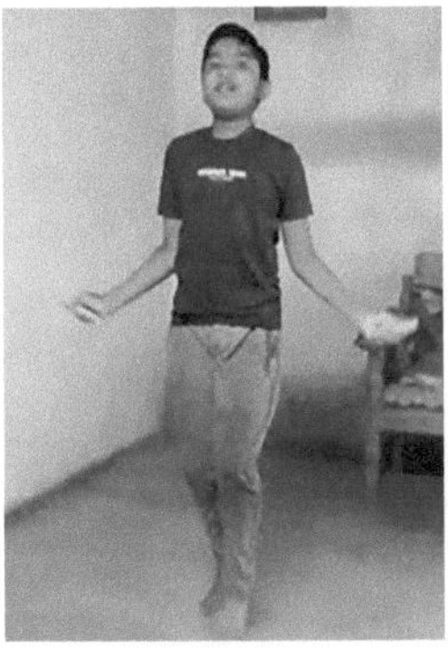
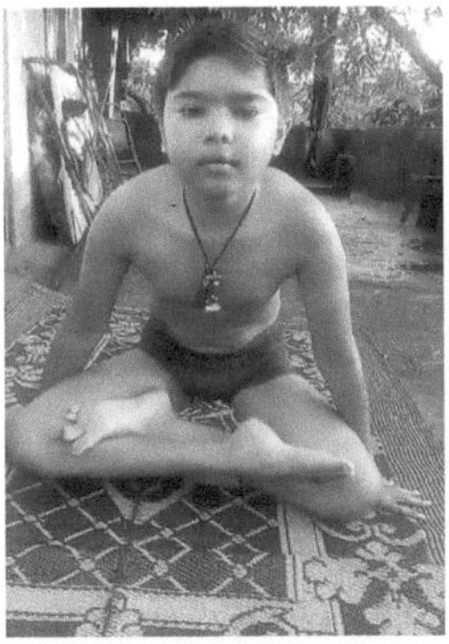
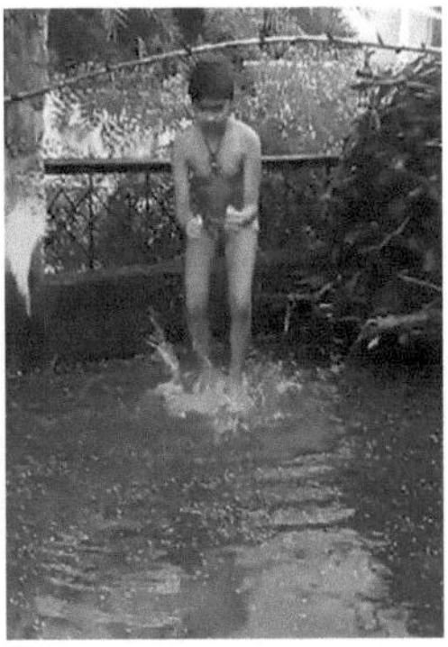
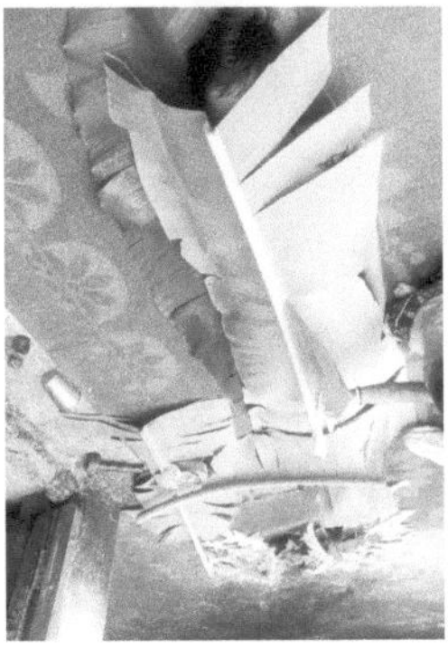
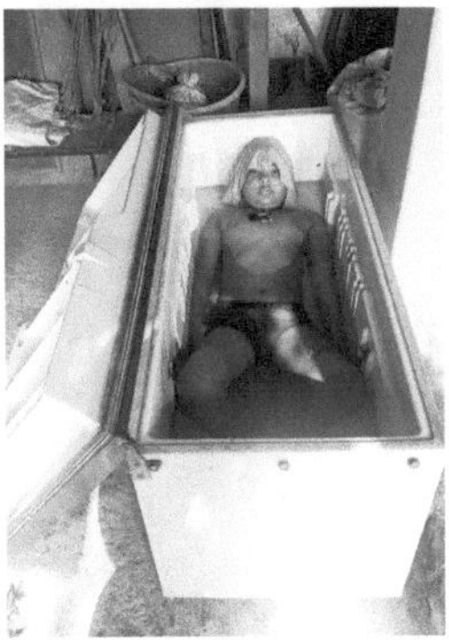
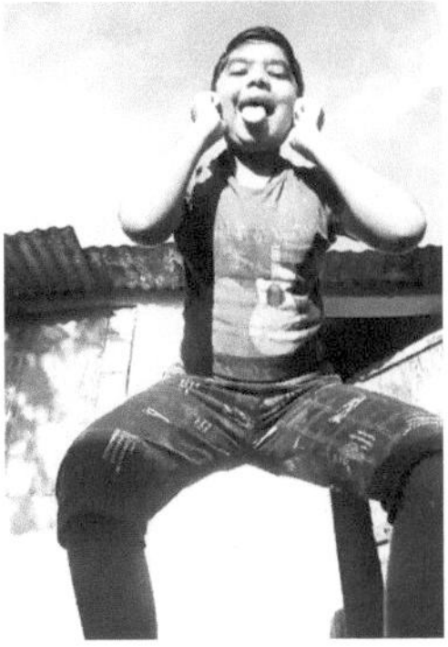

Following were Dev Kashyap parameters before starting Living Water Therapy:

**Frequency of transfusion:** once in 2 - 3 weeks

**Lowest Hemoglobin/ Hb ever recorded:** 4.2

**Medication taken:** Conimune, Danozen, Checal D, Folvite, Limce , Cetile, Protein, Trombopag, Rablet

**Physical Symptoms /Discomforts:** No discomforts

They came into our contact on 28- Jul-2022 and started Living Water Therapy.

The present status after starting the therapy

**Frequency of Transfusion:** Nil

**Medications:** Nil

**Physical Symptoms/ Discomforts:** Nil

*Uncle remarks, "my nephew has recovered so much that looking at him I can see him 80% cured. You have given us a simple way to cure this dreaded disease."*

# 14

Susil Kumar Barik age 10 years, son of Niranjan Barik(a trader by profession) and mother Mitashree Barik ( a homemaker), resides in Bhubaneswar, Odisha. Susil Kumar Barik was diagnosed with thalassemia for the first time at the age of 6 month. Just before the diagnosis he had crying most of the time. Doctor advised to go for blood test and that was the first time thalassemia was diagnosed. Since then he has been taking treatment at Capital Hospital Bhubaneswar.

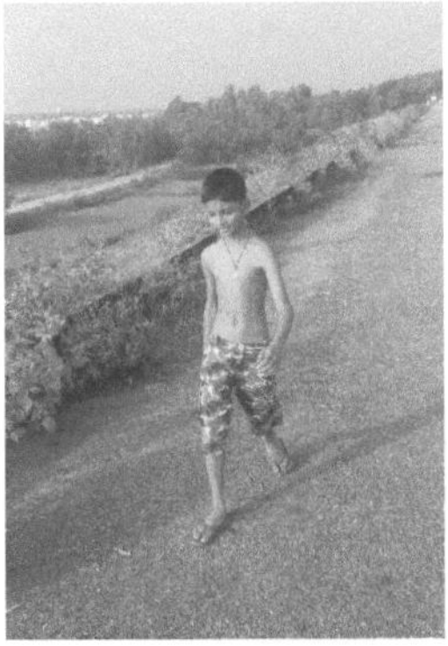

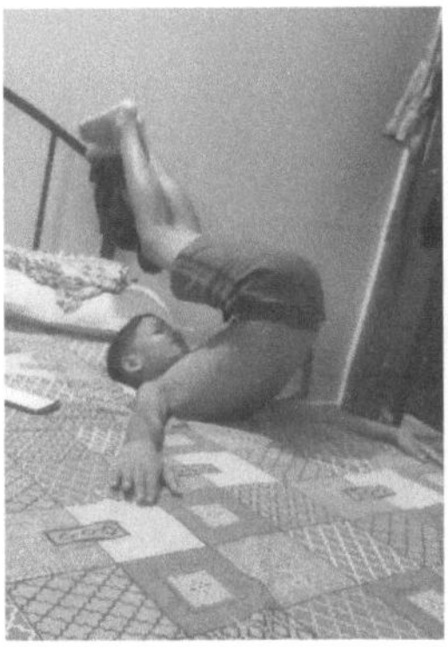

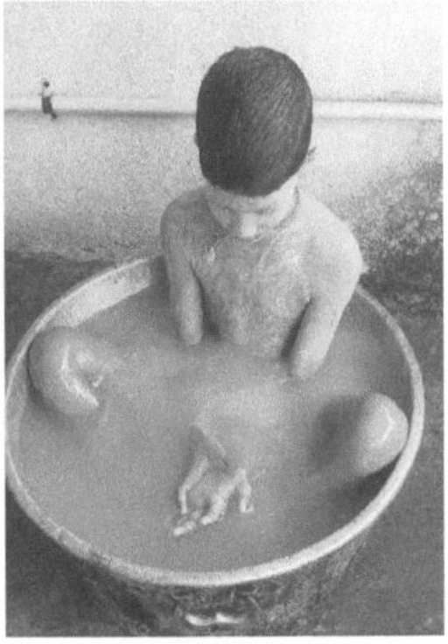

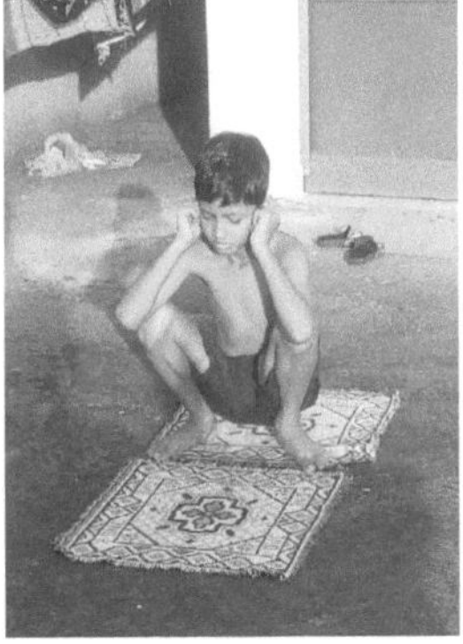

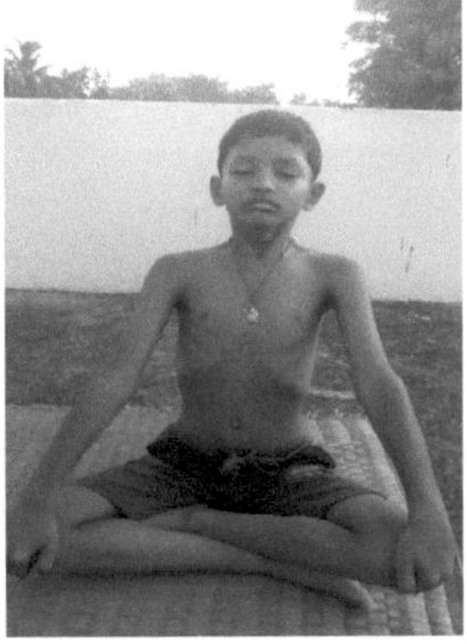

Following were Susil Kumar Barik parameters before starting Living Water Therapy:

**Frequency of transfusion:** once in 20 days

**Lowest Hemoglobin/ Hb ever recorded:** 7

**Medication taken:** Deferox

**Physical Symptoms /Discomforts:** Pale/ white body

They came into our contact on 30-Jul-2022 and started Living Water Therapy.

The present status after starting the therapy

**Frequency of Transfusion:** Nil

**Medications:** Nil

**Physical Symptoms/ Discomforts:** Nil

*Father's feedback, "In 20 days, our child is recovering quite well and I am feeling relaxed and very hopeful about my child's future."*

# 15

Harsh Raj age 11years, son of Sanjay Kumar( Special Warden at Central Jail Bhagalpur Bihar) and mother Bibha Kumari ( a homemaker), resides in Bhagalpur, Bihar. Harsh Raj was diagnosed with thalassemia for the first time at the age of 8 month. Just before the diagnosis he had weakness. Doctor advised to go for blood test and that was the first time thalassemia was diagnosed. Since then he has been taking treatment.

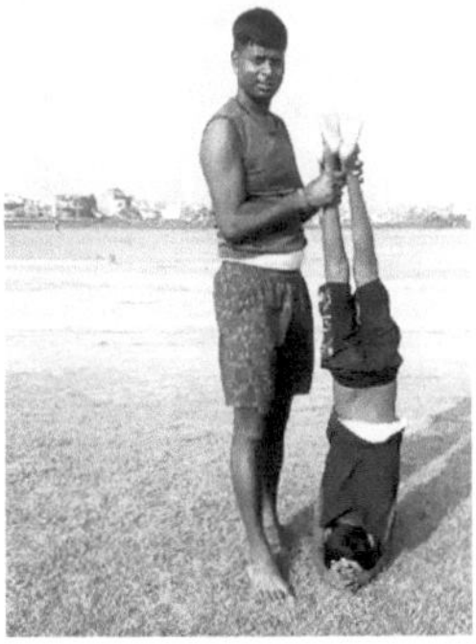

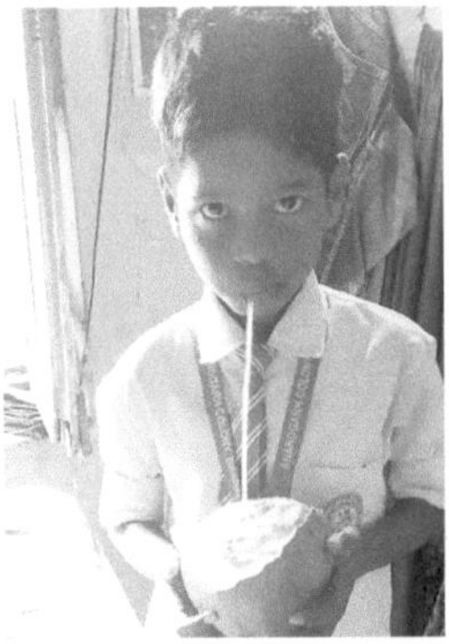

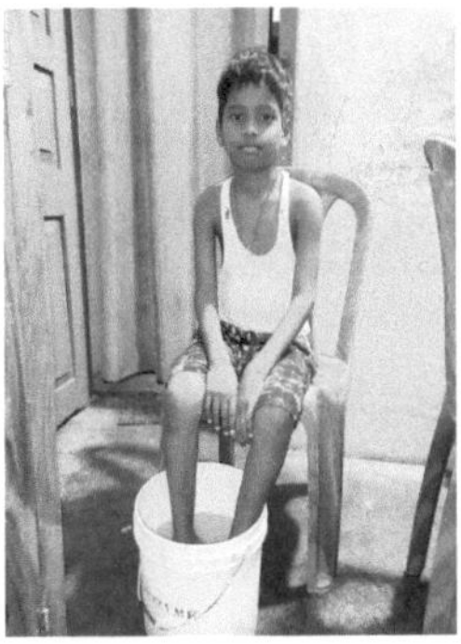

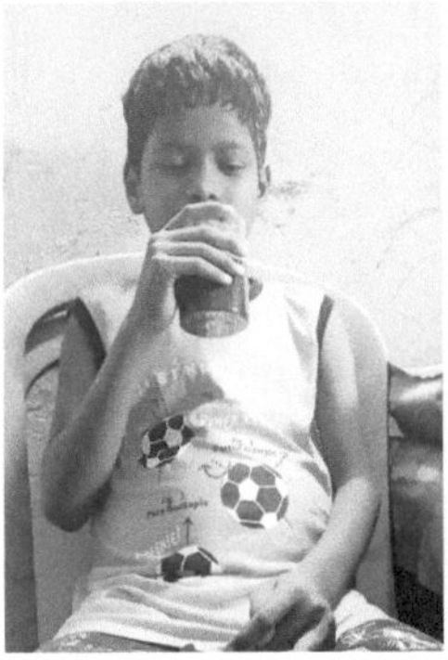

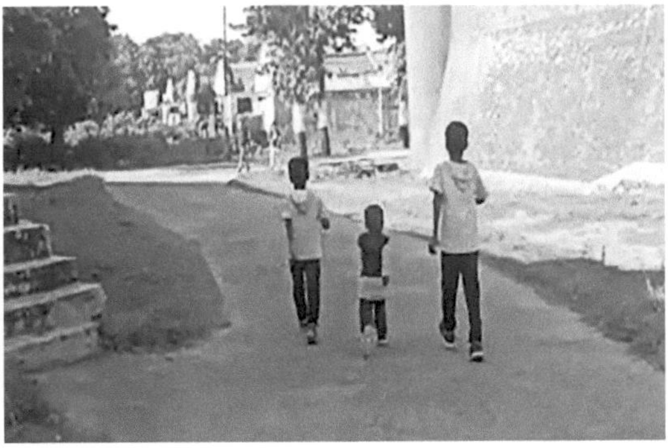

Following were Harsh Raj parameters before starting Living Water Therapy:

**Lowest Hemoglobin/ Hb ever recorded:** 4

**Medication taken:** Desirox 500mg

**Physical Symptoms /Discomforts:** Headache, loose motion, weakness

They came into our contact on 21-Jul-22 and started Living Water Therapy.

The present status after starting the therapy

**Medications:** Nil

**Physical Symptoms/ Discomforts:** Nil

*Harsh's father shares, "We almost died when our child was diagnosed with thalassemia. Relatives and friends who knew nothing about this disease were showering all kinds of advice on us. Little did they know how painful it was for the child and for us as parents? I don't know Dr BRC personally but what I do know is he has given us our life back. He is sent by God to help us pull out through this difficult time when all our near & dears failed to do so."*

# 16

Ruhan Gulam Mushtaq age 16 years, son of Gulam Mushtaq(a Self Employed) and mother Gulam Nilofar ( a homemaker), resides in Shrirampur, Maharashtra. Ruhan Gulam Mushtaq was diagnosed with thalassemia for the first time at the age of 15 years. Just before the diagnosis he had weakness. Doctor advised to go for blood test and that was the first time thalassemia was diagnosed. Since then he has been taking treatment at Chothani Hospital Srirampur.

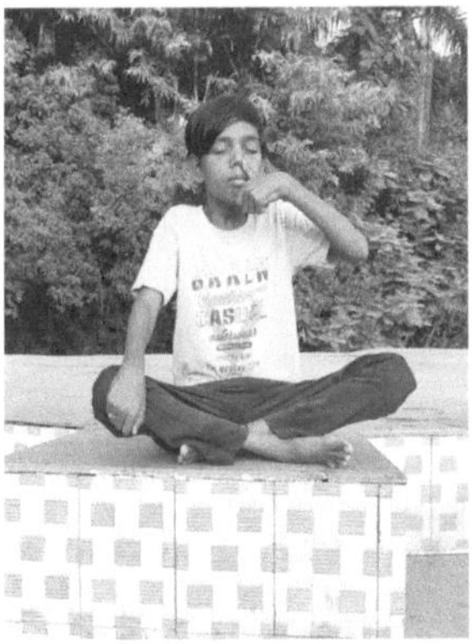
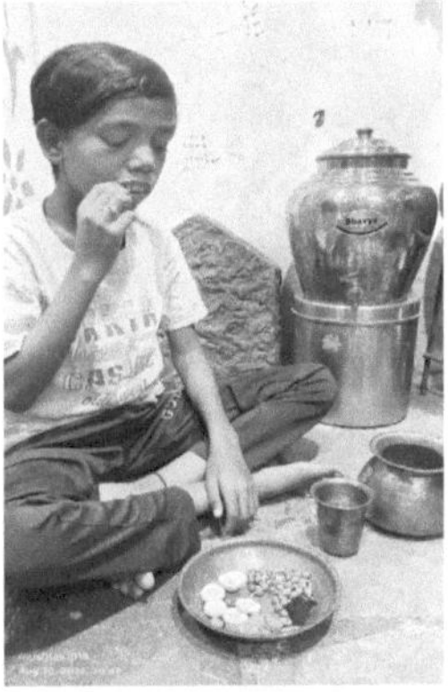
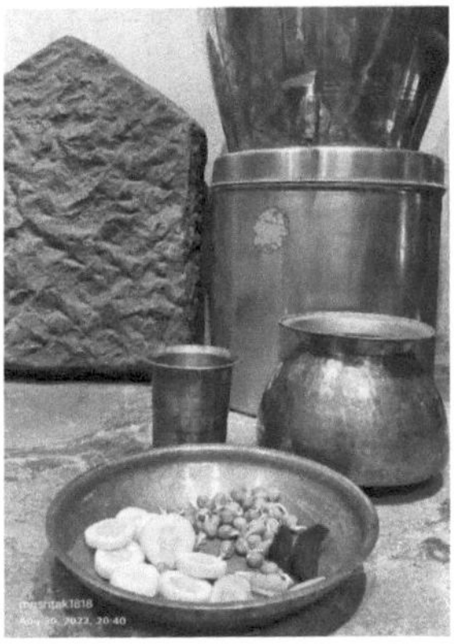
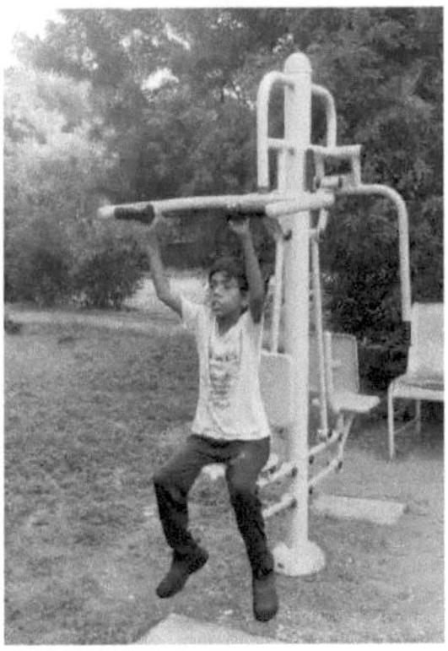

Following were Ruhan Gulam Mushtaq parameters before starting Living Water Therapy:

**Frequency of transfusion:** Twice a month

**Lowest Hemoglobin/ Hb ever recorded:** 4

**Physical Symptoms /Discomforts:** Weakness

They came into our contact on 20-Aug-22 and started Living Water Therapy.

The present status after starting the therapy

**Frequency of Transfusion:** Nil

**Physical Symptoms/ Discomforts:** Nil

# 17

Piyush age 15 years, son of Vinodbhai (a Gharkam) and mother Nutan (a homemaker), resides in Surat, Surat. Piyush was diagnosed with thalassemia for the first time at the age of 2 years. Just before the diagnosis he had consistent fever and pale skin/body. Doctor advised to go for blood test and that was the first time thalassemia was diagnosed. Since then he has been taking treatment at Bhavnagar Civil Hospital.

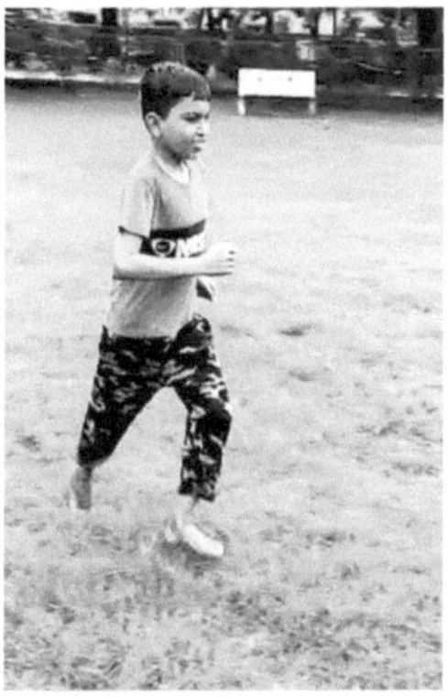
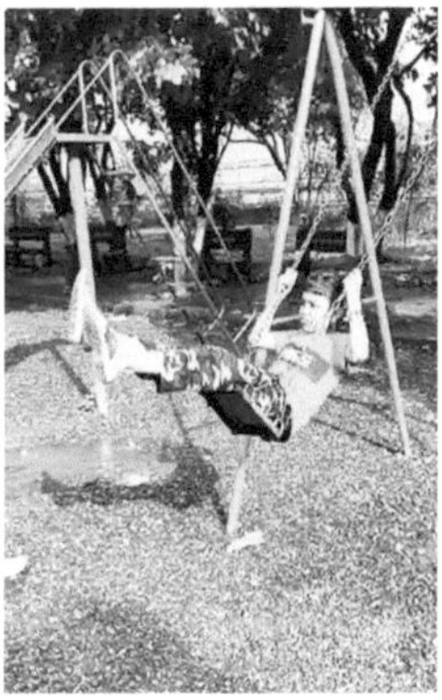
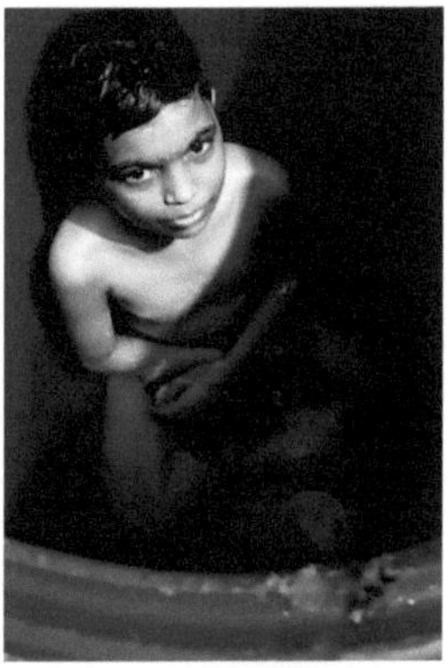
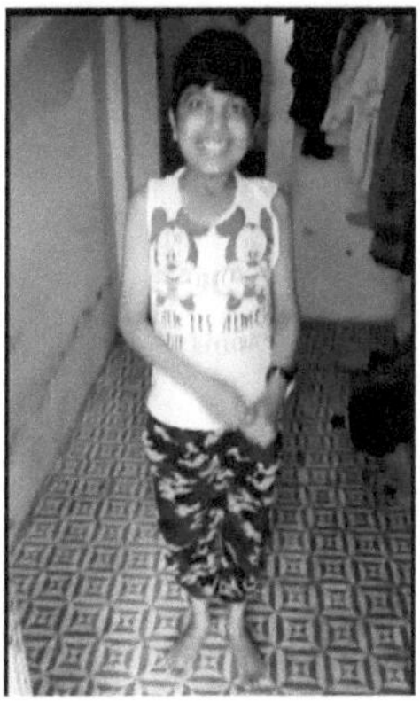
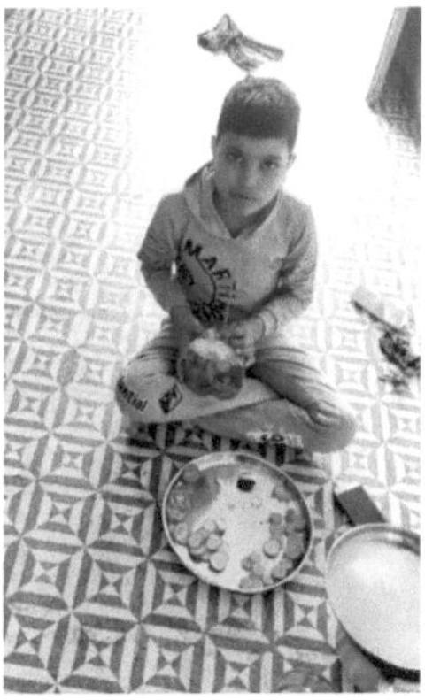
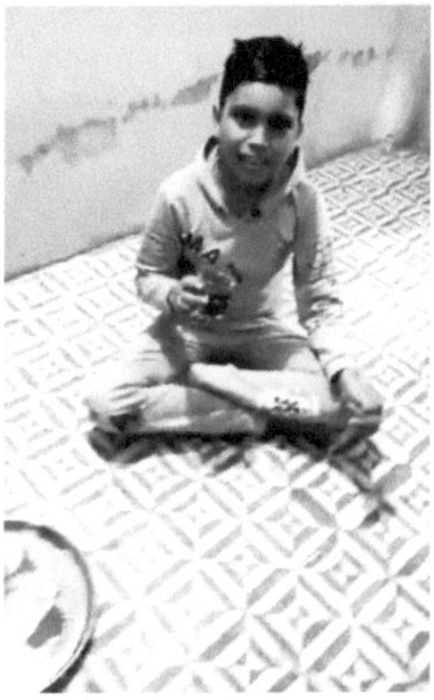

Following were Piyush parameters before starting Living Water Therapy:

**Frequency of transfusion:** twice a month

**Lowest Hemoglobin/ Hb ever recorded:** 6

**Medication taken:** Deferasirox,folic acid , Becostal

**Physical Symptoms /Discomforts:** Weakness and pain in legs

They came into our contact on 7-Aug- 2022 and started Living Water Therapy.

The present status after starting the therapy

**Frequency of Transfusion:** Nil

**Medications:** Nil

**Physical Symptoms/ Discomforts:** Nil

# 18

Aafiya age 6.5 yrs, daughter of Ali Akbar (owns a furniture shop) and mother Yasmeen Galaria ( a homemaker), resides in Asansol, West bengal. Aafiya was diagnosed with thalassemia for the first time at the age of 7 months. Just before the diagnosis she had loose motion. Doctor advised to go for blood test and that was the first time thalassemia was diagnosed. Since then she has been taking treatment at Bhoruka Transfusion center.

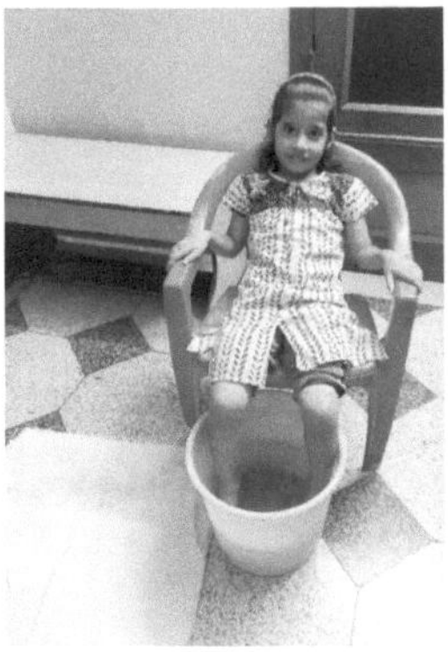

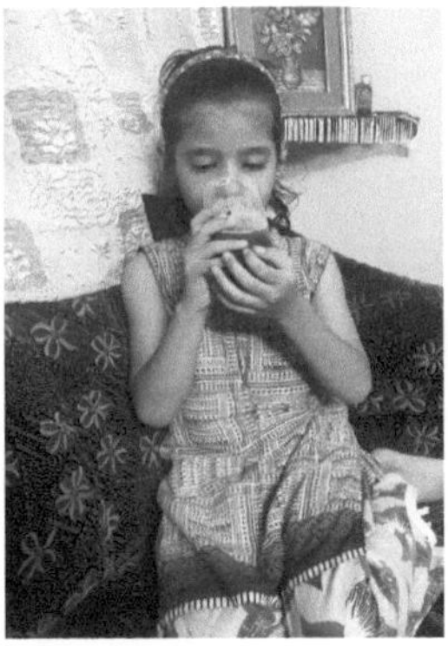

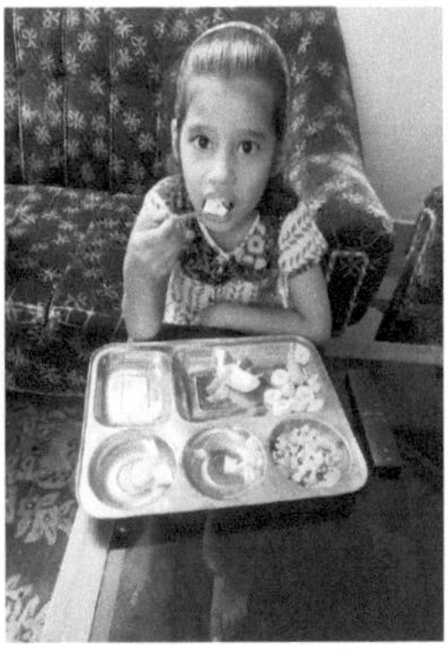

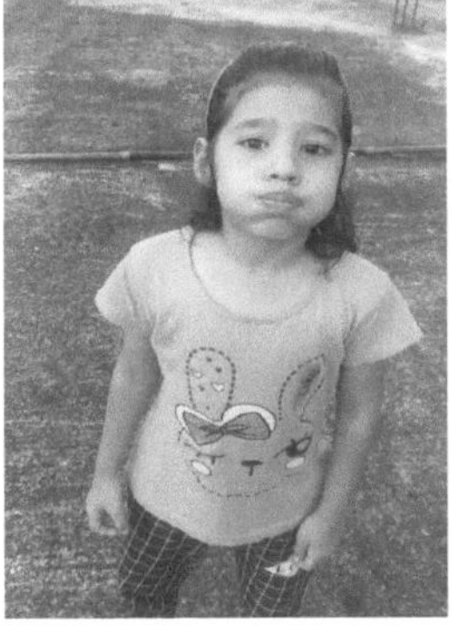

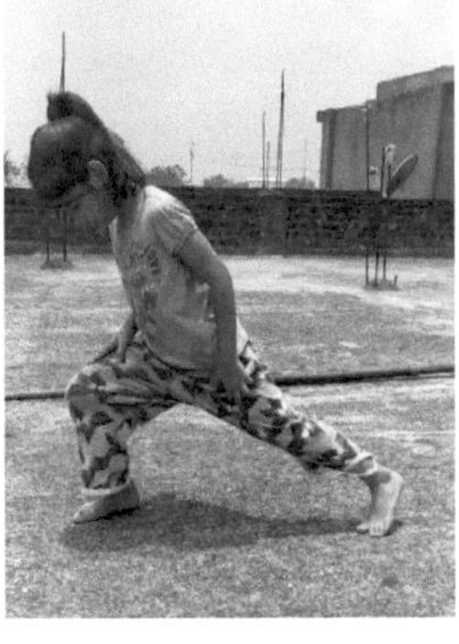

Following were Aafiya parameters before starting Living Water Therapy:

**Frequency of transfusion:** once in 21 days

**Lowest Hemoglobin/ Hb ever recorded:** 8

**Medication taken:** Folvite, Evion LC,Defrijet.

**Physical Symptoms /Discomforts:** Restless sleep,becomes angry, and doesn't want to eat.

They came into our contact on 25-Jul-22 and started Living Water Therapy.

The present status after starting the therapy

**Frequency of Transfusion:** Nil

**Medications:** Nil

**Physical Symptoms/ Discomforts:** Nil

*A Happy father announces, "My daughter loves and likes to follow Living Water Therapy, be it food, drawing, walking on grass, climbing trees, exercise. You name it, she loves all!"*

# 19

Divyansh Namdev age 9 years, son of Hariom Namdev (a tailor) and mother Mamta Namdev ( a homemaker), resides in Vidisha, M.P. Divyansh Namdev was diagnosed with thalassemia for the first time at the age of 6 month. Just before the diagnosis he had high fever. Doctor advised to go for blood test and that was the first time thalassemia was diagnosed. Since then he has been taking treatment at District Hospital Vidisha Madhya Pradesh.

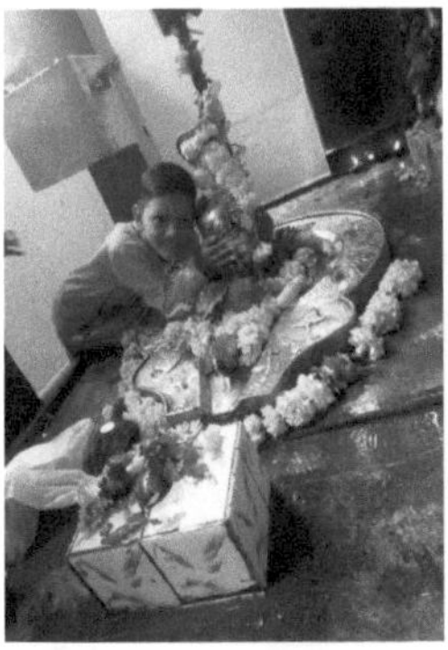
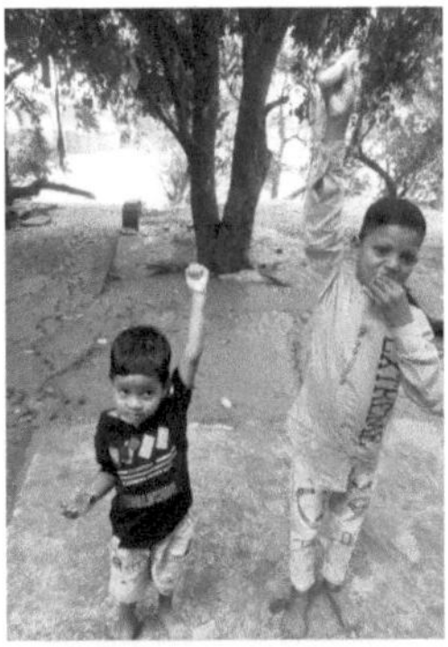
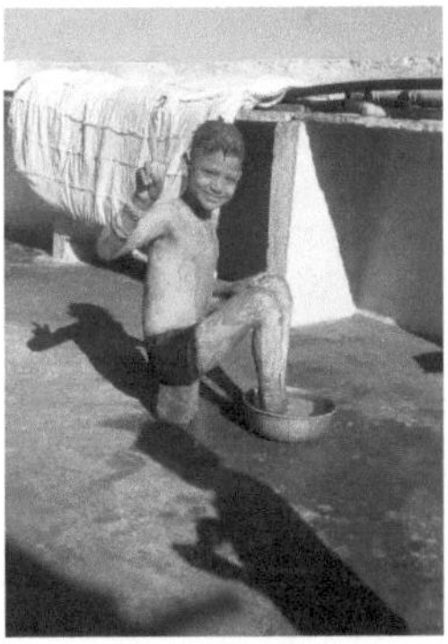
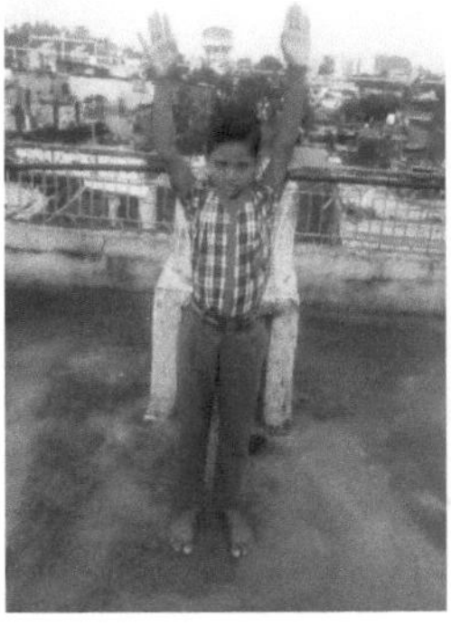
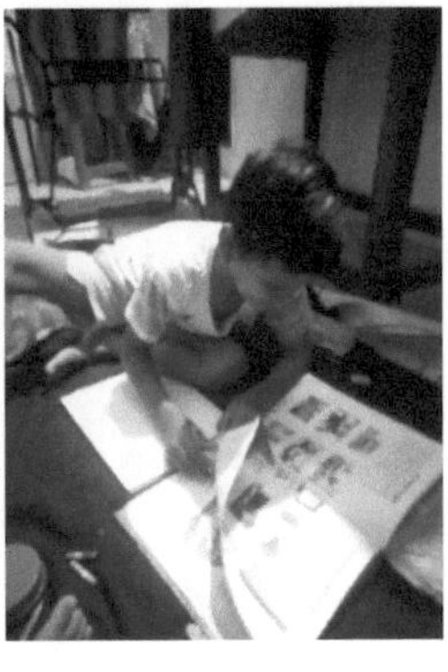
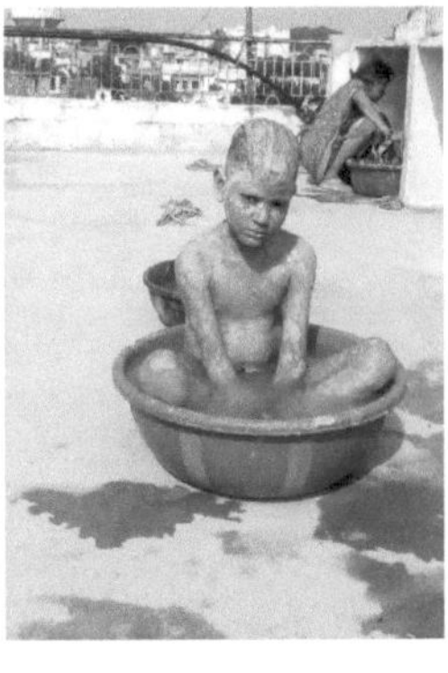

Following were Divyansh Namdev parameters before starting Living Water Therapy:

**Frequency of transfusion:** twice a month

**Lowest Hemoglobin/ Hb ever recorded:** 8

**Medication taken:** Folic acid desiroks

**Physical Symptoms /Discomforts:** High fever

They came into our contact on 25-Jul-2022 and started Living Water Therapy.

The present status after starting the therapy

**Frequency of Transfusion:** Nil

**Medications:** Nil

**Physical Symptoms/ Discomforts:** Nil

# 20

Mazhar Ali Baig age 16 years, son of Ashraf Ali Baig (a tailor) and mother Samina begum ( a homemaker), resides in Behram Nagar Bandra East Mumbai, Maharashtra. Mazhar Ali Baig was diagnosed with thalassemia for the first time at the age of 4 months. Just before the diagnosis he had high fever. Doctor advised to go for blood test and that was the first time thalassemia was diagnosed. Since then he has been taking treatment at Yashoda Hospital Pune.

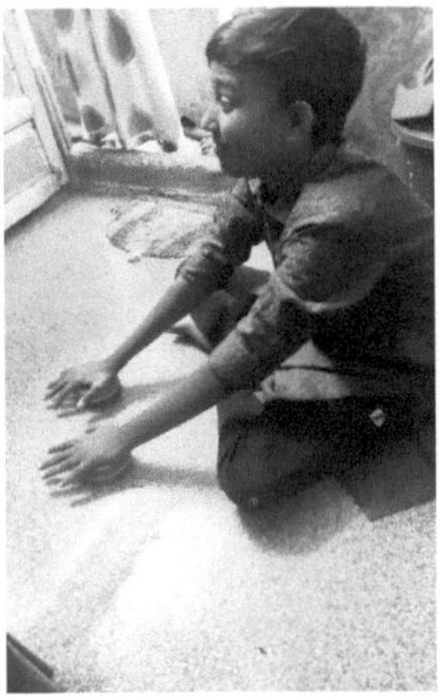
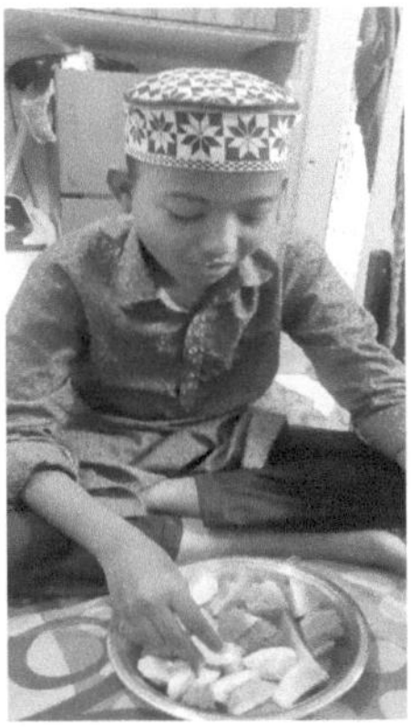
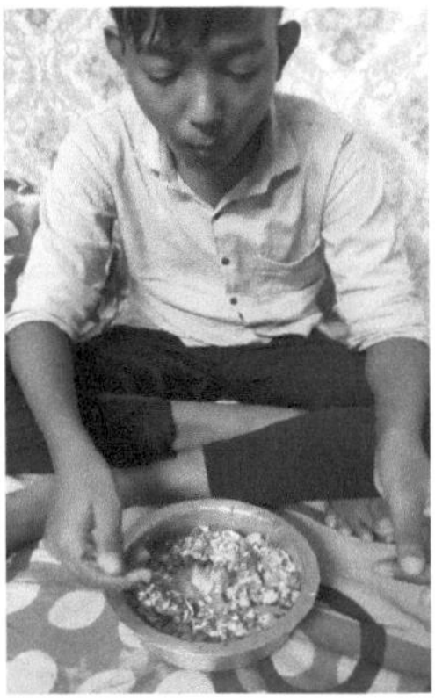
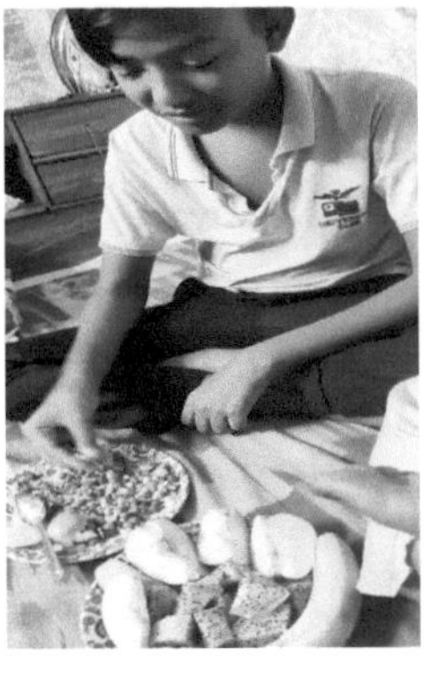
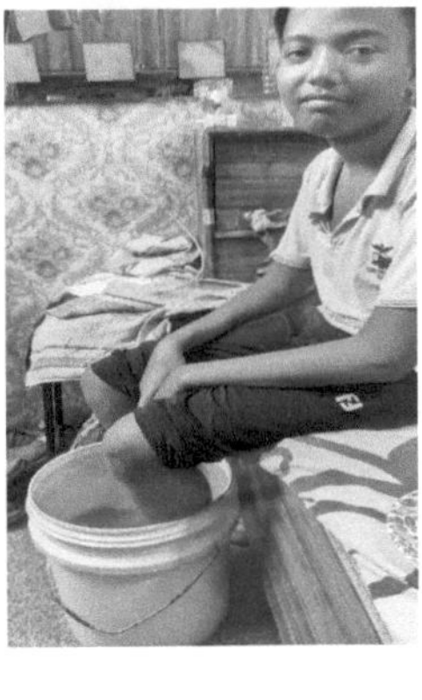

Following were Mazhar Ali Baig parameters before starting Living Water Therapy:

**Frequency of transfusion:** once in 6 months only if required

**Lowest Hemoglobin/ Hb ever recorded:** 5.2

**Medication taken:** Thalidomide, Ubilife, Sapsure, Glutaone

**Physical Symptoms /Discomforts:** Weakness, high heart rate, problem in long distance walking

They came into our contact on 29-Jul-2022 and started Living Water Therapy.

The present status after starting the therapy

**Frequency of Transfusion:** Nil

**Medications:** Nil

**Physical Symptoms/ Discomforts:** Nil

*Father's feedback, "For the sake of the children this program (Living Water Therapy) should continue*

# 21

Rohan Naik age 10 years, son of Umakanta Naik (a two wheeler mechanic) and mother Babita naik (a homemaker), resides in Bolangir, Odissa. Rohan Naik was diagnosed with thalassemia for the first time at the age of 6 months. Just before the diagnosis he had consistent fever. Doctor advised to go for blood test and that was the first time thalassemia was diagnosed. Since then he has been taking treatment at AIIMS Hospital Bhubaneshwar.

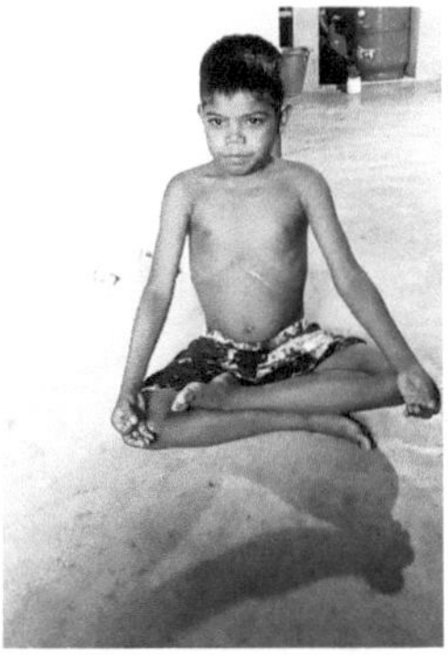

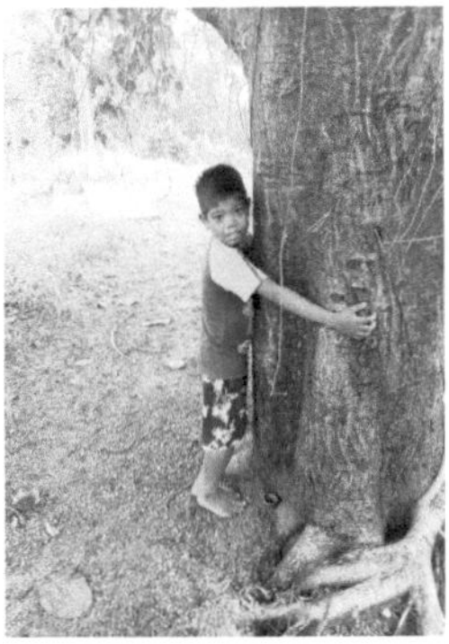

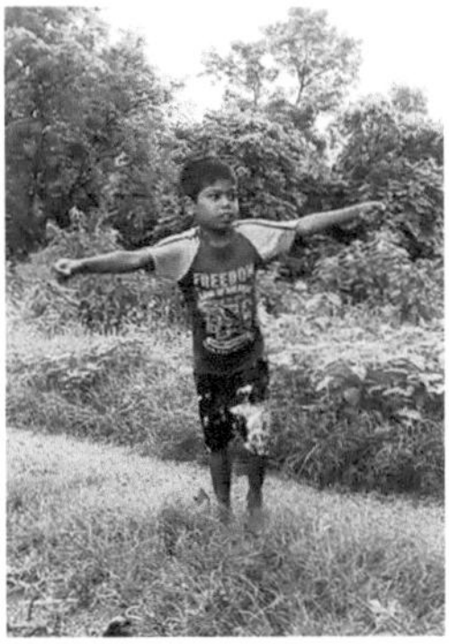

Following were Rohan Naik parameters before starting Living Water Therapy:

**Frequency of transfusion:** once a month

**Lowest Hemoglobin/ Hb ever recorded:** 4

**Medication taken:** Folic acid,dosider,durea

**Physical Symptoms /Discomforts:** Nil

They came into our contact on 21-Jul-2022 and started Living Water Therapy.

The present status after starting the therapy

**Frequency of Transfusion:** Nil

**Medications:** Nil

**Physical Symptoms/ Discomforts:** Nil

*Thankful father remarks, "Ever since the program started we have not gone for transfusion at all, neither we want to. Things are going very well and am sure that positive results will continue. Thanks to Dr BRC and Dr Namita."*

# 22

Piyush Sonkar age 4 years, son of Kanhiya Sonkar(a fruit whole-seller) and mother Riya Sonkar ( a homemaker), resides in Rudrapur (Devoriya), Uttar Pradesh. Piyush Sonkar was diagnosed with thalassemia for the first time at the age of 2 months. Just before the diagnosis he used to continuously cry all the time. Doctor advised to go for blood test and that was the first time thalassemia was diagnosed. Since then he has been taking treatment at Gorakhpur.

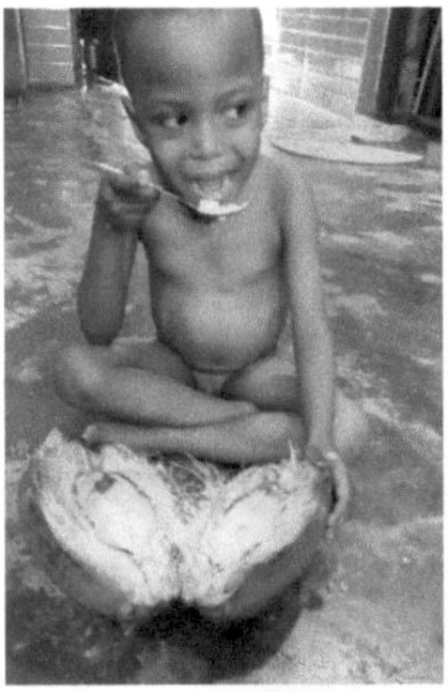
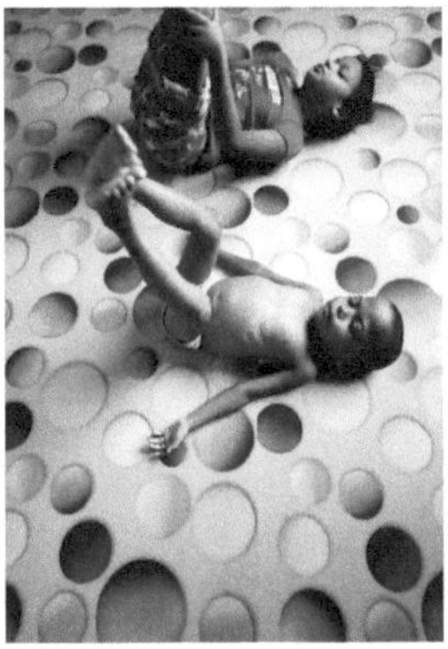
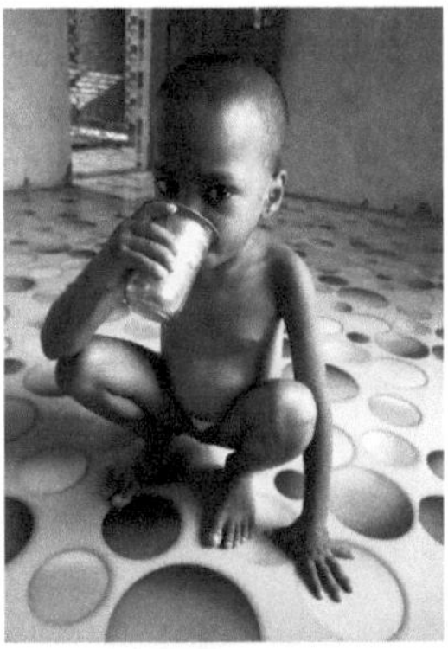
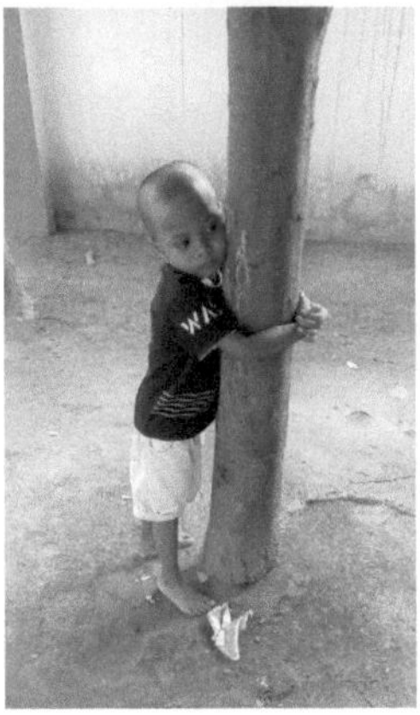
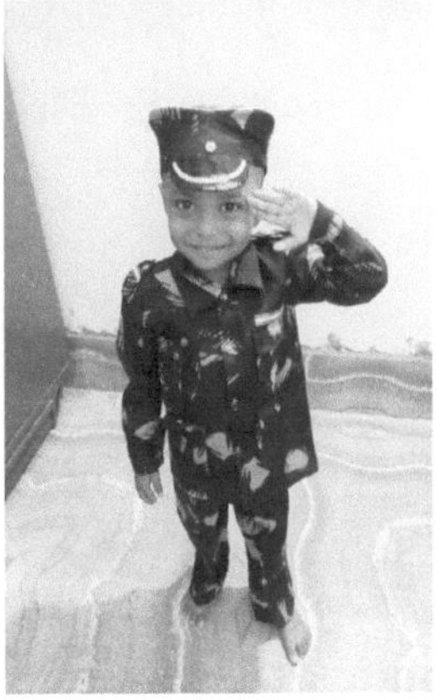
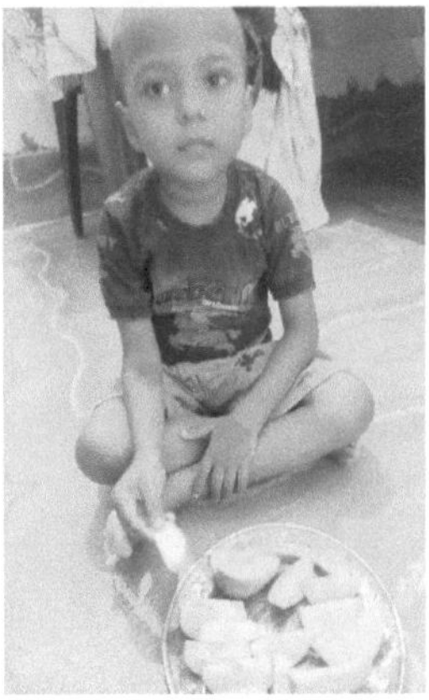

Following were Piyush Sonkar parameters before starting Living Water Therapy:

Frequency of transfusion: once in 25 days

**Lowest Hemoglobin/ Hb ever recorded:** 4

**Medication taken:** Folic acid

**Physical Symptoms /Discomforts:** fever and body skin gets yellow

They came into our contact on 31-Jul-2022 and started Living Water Therapy.

The present status after starting the therapy

**Frequency of Transfusion:** Nil:

**Medications:** Nil

**Physical Symptoms/ Discomforts:** Nil

*Father shares, "I was fed up of going to big hospitals looking for a cure for my child. But now I have stopped that ever since we started Living Water Therapy. Not only my child but even I am following the same protocol. I have also recovered with my son. My kid looks all pink and red. I am avoiding going to labs for blood tests as I can see the results crystal clear."*

# 23

Jeet Adhikary age 17 years, son of Achintya Adhikary (a runs his own business) and mother Durga Adhikary (a homemaker), resides in Kolkata, West Bengal. Jeet Adhikary was diagnosed with thalassemia for the first time at the age of 3 months. Just before the diagnosis he was refusing to eat food. Doctor advised to go for blood test and that was the first time thalassemia was diagnosed. Since then he has been taking treatment at Indian Association of Blood Cancer & Diagnosis Centre.

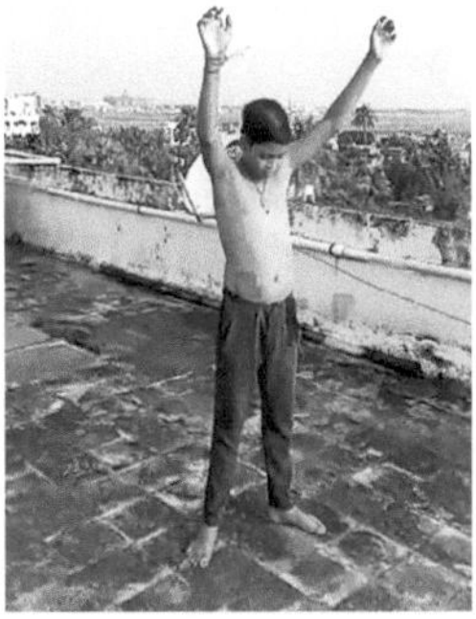
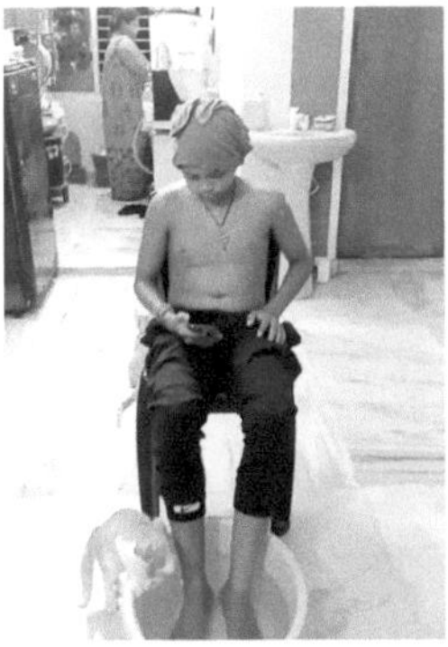
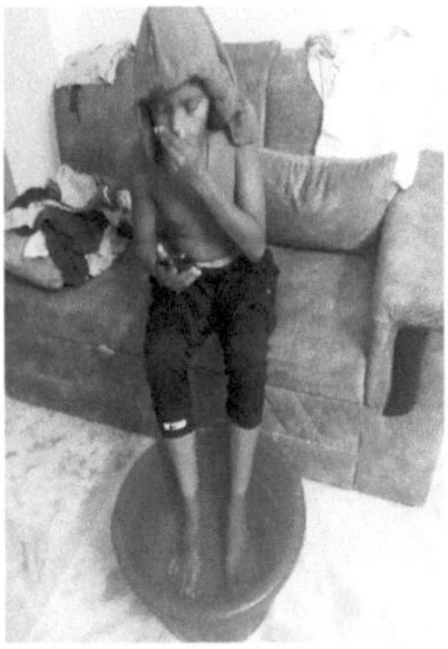
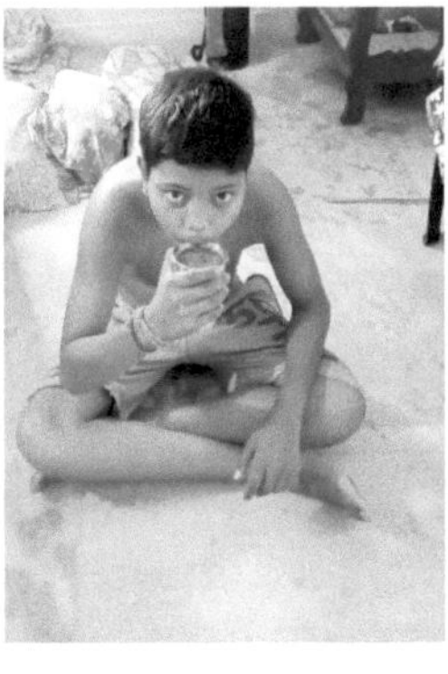
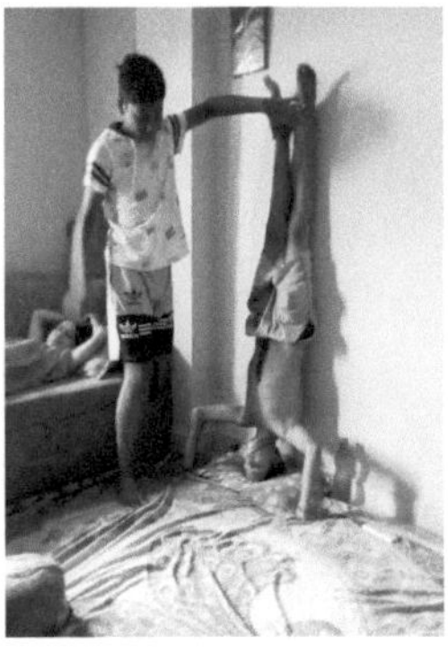
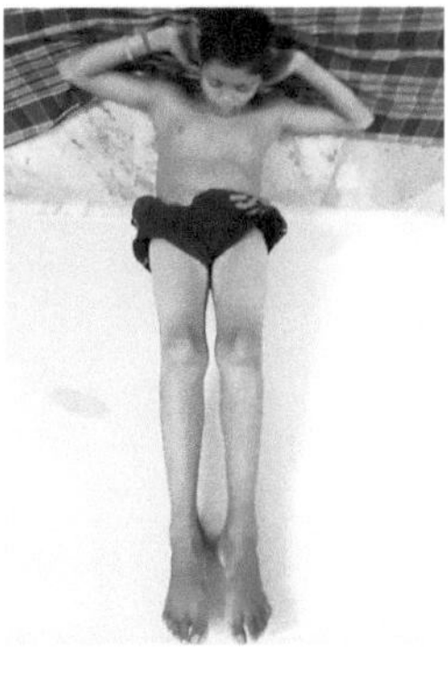

Following were Jeet Adhikary parameters before starting Living Water Therapy:

**Frequency of transfusion:** 4-5 times in a month

**Lowest Hemoglobin/ Hb ever recorded:** 5.5

**Medication taken:** Kelfer

**Physical Symptoms /Discomforts:** Headache and breathing problem

They came into our contact on 27-Jul-2022 and started Living Water Therapy.

The present status after starting the therapy

**Frequency of Transfusion:** Nil

**Medications:** Nil

**Physical Symptoms/ Discomforts:** Nil

*Jeet shares, "I am very healthy with Living Water Therapy. I don't need transfusions now. Sometimes whenever I feel weak I follow all the protocol and recover quickly. Not only me but my whole family has benefitted following the protocol along with me."*

# 24

Sachi Vivek Wankhede age 3 years, daughter of Vivek Vishwanath Wankhede(works on daily wages) and mother Kalyani Vivek Wankhede ( a homemaker), resides in Nagpur, Maharashtra. Sachi Vivek Wankhede was diagnosed with thalassemia for the first time at the age of 18 months. Just before the diagnosis she had fever and stomach infection. Doctor advised to go for blood test and that was the first time thalassemia was diagnosed. Since then she has been taking treatment at Nucleous Hospital Nagpur.

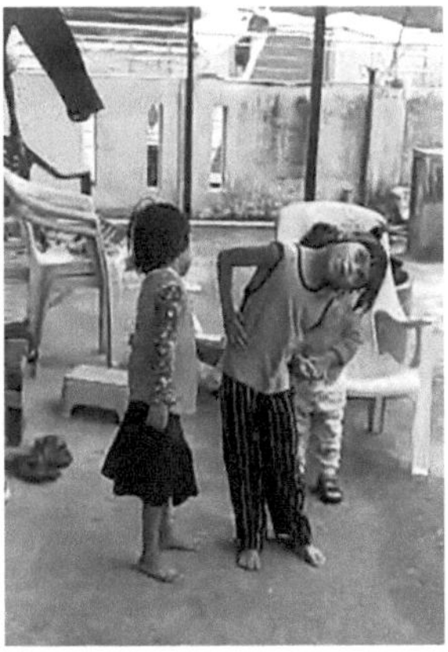

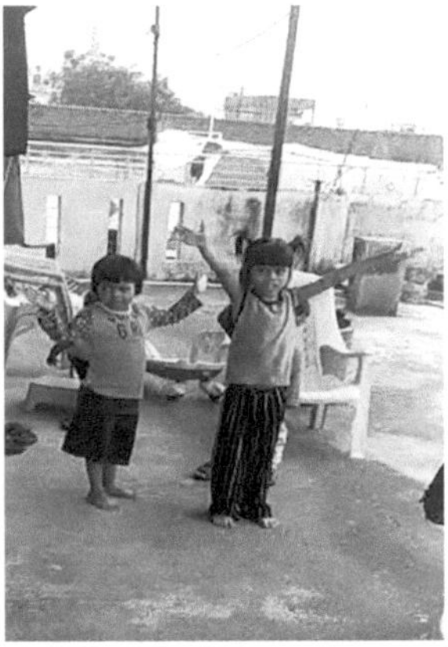

Following were Sachi Vivek Wankhede parameters before starting Living Water Therapy:

**Frequency of transfusion:** once a year

**Lowest Hemoglobin/ Hb ever recorded:** 3.2

**Medication taken:** Folic acid and zincovit syrup

**Physical Symptoms /Discomforts:** Fever and stomach infection and yellow body colour

They came into our contact on 23-Jul-2022 and started Living Water Therapy.

The present status after starting the therapy

**Frequency of Transfusion:** Nil

**Medications:** Nil

**Physical Symptoms/ Discomforts:** Nil

# 25

Jiniya Vivek Wankhede, age 6 years, daughter of Vivek Vishwanath Wankhede (works on daily wages) and mother Kalyani Vivek Wankhede (a homemaker), resides in Nagpur, Maharashtra. Jiniya Vivek Wankhede was diagnosed with thalassemia for the first time at the age of 5 years. Just before the diagnosis she had Fever. Doctor advised to go for blood test and that was the first time thalassemia was diagnosed. Since then she has been taking treatment at Government Medical College.

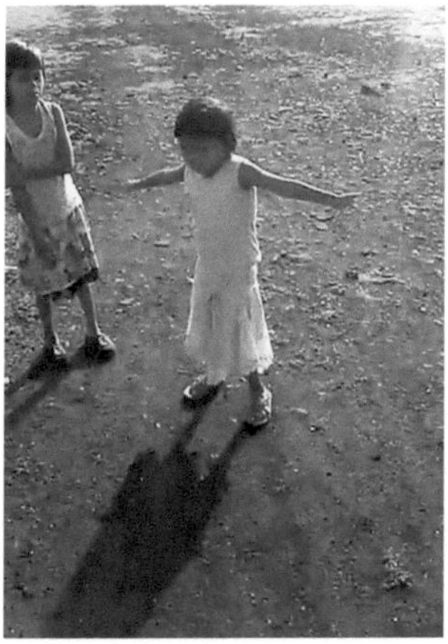

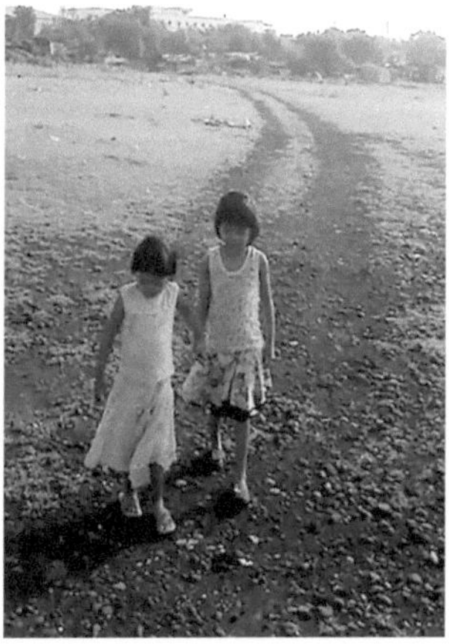

Following were Jiniya Vivek Wankhede parameters before starting Living Water Therapy:

**Frequency of transfusion:** only once till now

**Lowest Hemoglobin/ Hb ever recorded:** 4.7

**Medication taken:** Folic Acid and Zincovit

**Physical Symptoms /Discomforts:** Fever and Joint pain

They came into our contact on 23-Jul-2022 and started Living Water Therapy.

The present status after starting the therapy

**Frequency of Transfusion:** Nil

**Medications:** Nil

**Physical Symptoms/ Discomforts:** Nil

# 26

Vaidahi Shankarrao Aragade age 7 years, daughter of Shankarrao Nivrutti Aragade (runs his own business) and mother Supriya Shankarrao Aragade (a homemaker), resides in Ichalkaranji, Maharashtra. Vaidahi Shankarrao Aragade was diagnosed with thalassemia for the first time at the age of 4 month. Just before the diagnosis she had weakness. Doctor advised to go for blood test and that was the first time thalassemia was diagnosed. Since then she has been taking treatment at Asha Bal and Netra Hospital.

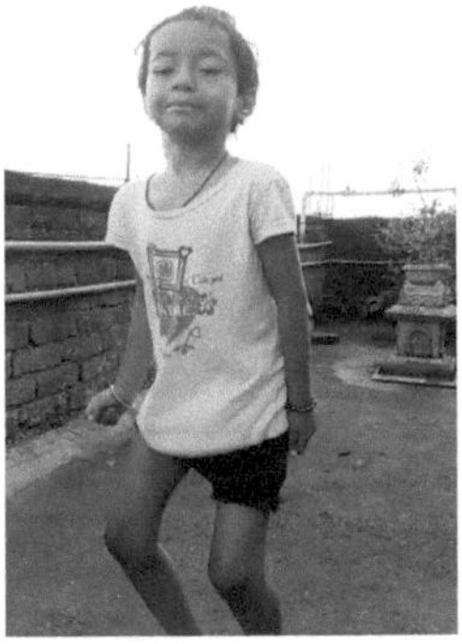

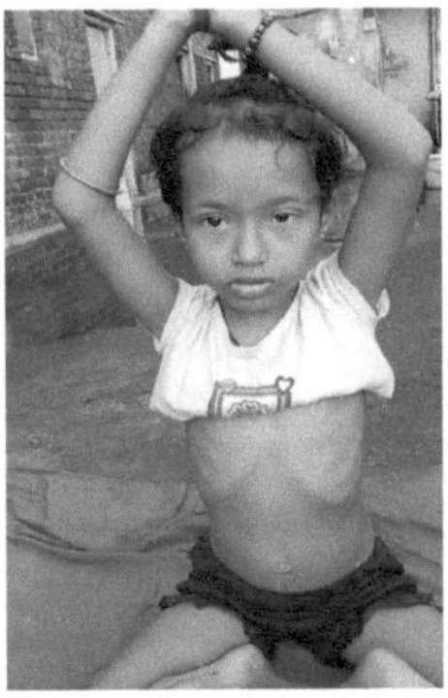

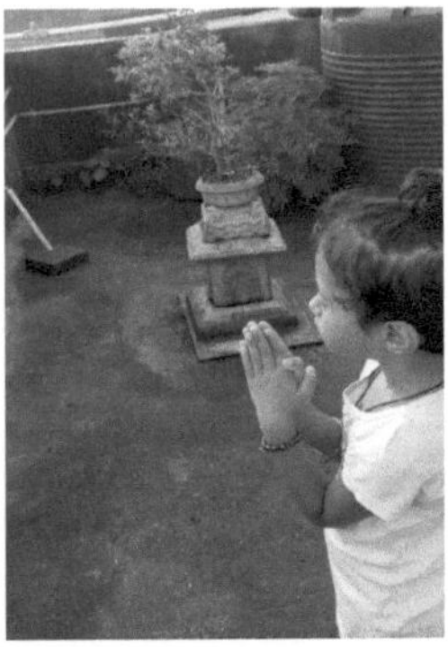

Following were Vaidahi Shankarrao Aragade parameters before starting Living Water Therapy:

**Frequency of transfusion:** once a month

**Lowest Hemoglobin/ Hb ever recorded:** 4.2

**Medication taken:** Desirox 500 ,kelfer 250, fol 5, calcimax p, zincovit

**Physical Symptoms /Discomforts:** Energy down , face colour is yellow and white

They came into our contact on 20- Jul-2022 and started Living Water Therapy.

The present status after starting the therapy

**Frequency of Transfusion:** Nil

**Medications:** Nil

**Physical Symptoms/ Discomforts:** Nil

*Father shares, "My daughter has already defeated her disease. No more hospital & hospital beds for my child. Thanks to Dr BRC & Dr Namita."*

# 27

Lokesh Pramanik age 3.5 years, son of Praful Pramanik(a Service man) and mother Rupa Devi (a homemaker), resides in Dhanbad, Jharkhand. Lokesh Pramanik was diagnosed with thalassemia for the first time at the age of 2.5 months. Just before the diagnosis he had fever. Doctor advised to go for blood test and that was the first time thalassemia was diagnosed. Since then he has been taking treatment at CMC Vellore.

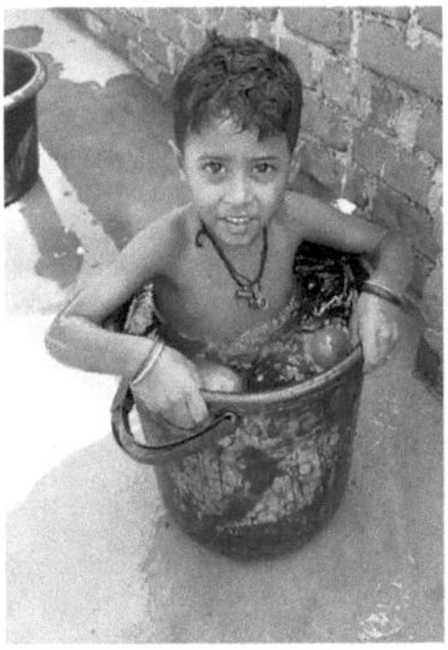
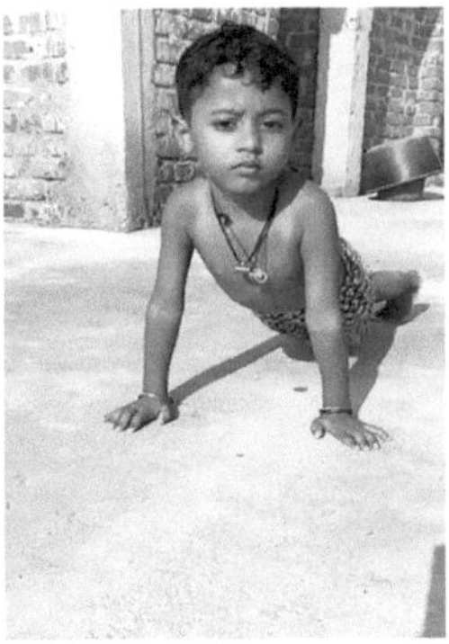
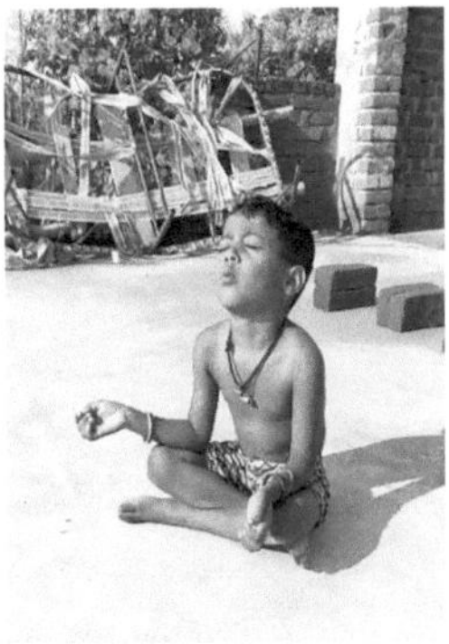

Following were Lokesh Pramanik parameters before starting Living Water Therapy:

**Frequency of transfusion:** once a month

**Lowest Hemoglobin/ Hb ever recorded:** 7

**Medication taken:** Folvite,Desirock500

**Physical Symptoms /Discomforts:** Nil

They came into our contact on 15-Aug-2022 and started Living Water Therapy.

The present status after starting the therapy

**Frequency of Transfusion:** Nil

**Medications:** Nil

**Physical Symptoms/ Discomforts:** Nil

# 28

Swikruti Ramchandra Kamble age 8 years, daughter of Ramchandra Krishnat Kamble (a farmer) and mother sarika (a homemaker), resides in kolhapur, Maharastra. Swikruti Ramchandra Kamble was diagnosed with thalassemia for the first time at the age of 5 month. Just before the diagnosis she had fever problem. Doctor advised to go for blood test and that was the first time thalassemia was diagnosed. Since then she has been taking treatment at Masai Hospital Kolhapur.

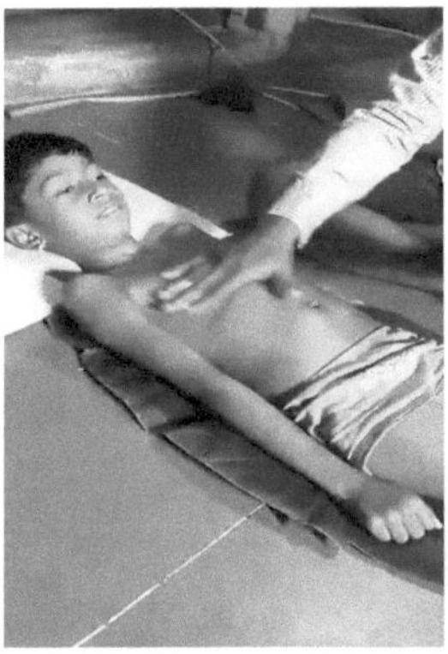

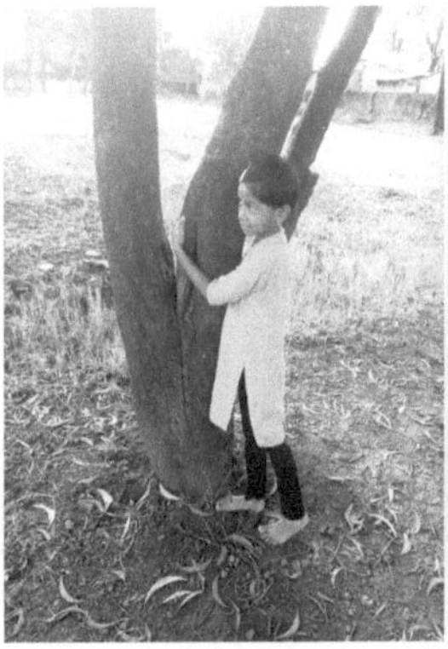

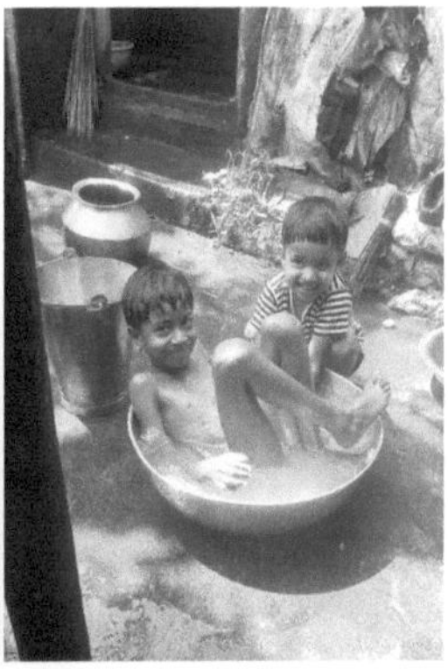

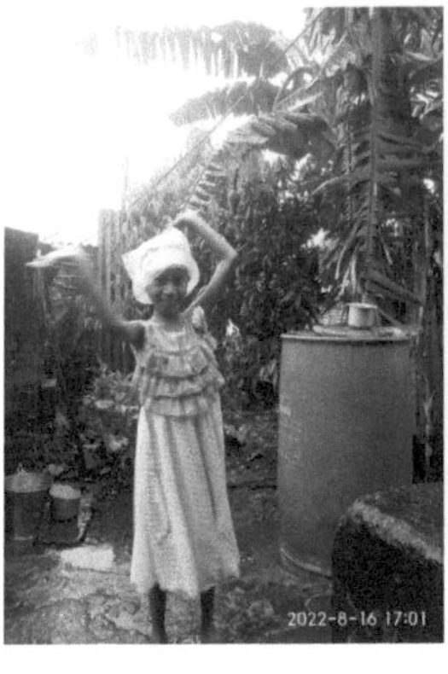


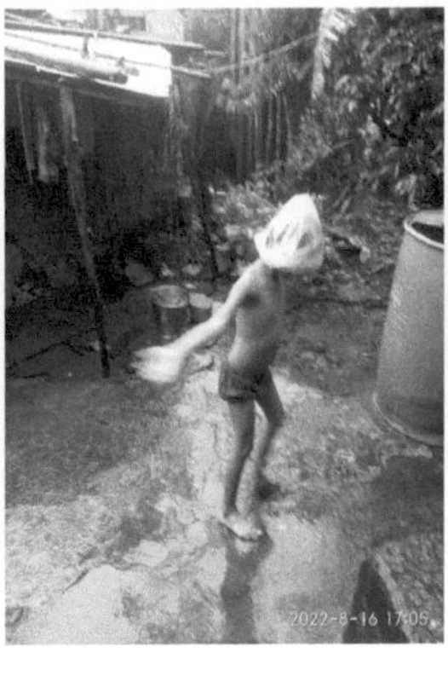


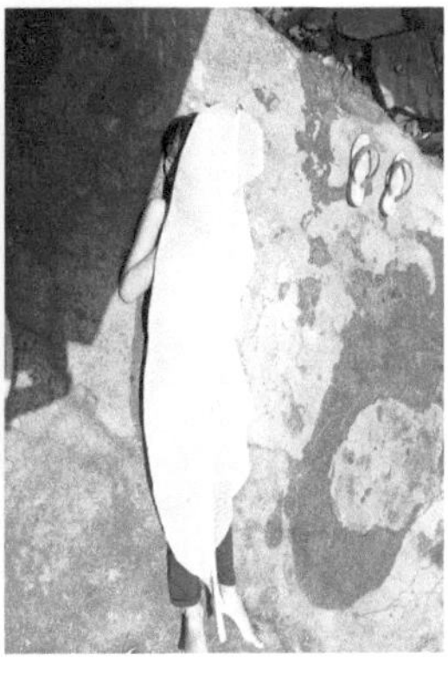

Following were Swikruti Ramchandra Kamble parameters before starting Living Water Therapy:

**Frequency of transfusion:** once a month

**Lowest Hemoglobin/ Hb ever recorded:** 7

**Medication taken:** desirox

**Physical Symptoms /Discomforts:** fever

They came into our contact on 23-Jul-2022 and started Living Water Therapy.

The present status after starting the therapy

**Frequency of Transfusion:** Nil

**Medications:** Nil

**Physical Symptoms/ Discomforts:** Nil

*Father remarks, "I meet so many patients in the hospital. After following Living Water Therapy, my daughter is totally healed .I will now connect with these patients n dedicate myself towards this noble cause bring awareness about DIP diet n Living Water Therapy."*

# 29

Sandeep Kumar Mohanty age 6 years, son of Prasant Kumar Mohanty (self employed) and mother Santosini Mohanty ( a homemaker), resides in Paralakhemundi, Odisha. Sandeep Kumar Mohanty was diagnosed with thalassemia for the first time at the age of 3 month. Just before the diagnosis parents observed his pale skin. Doctor advised to go for blood test and that was the first time thalassemia was diagnosed. Since then he has been taking treatment at DHH Paralakhemundi.

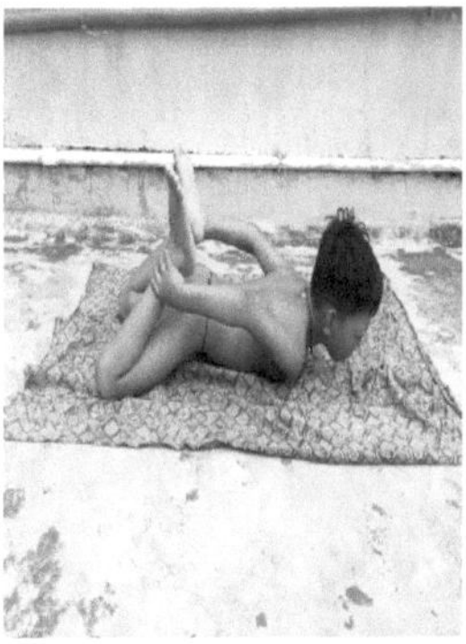
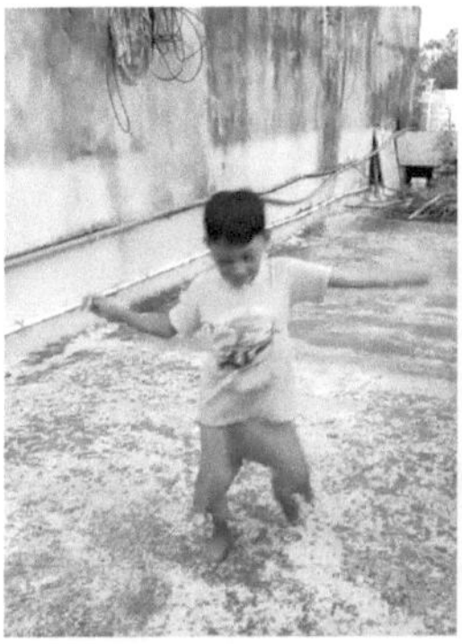
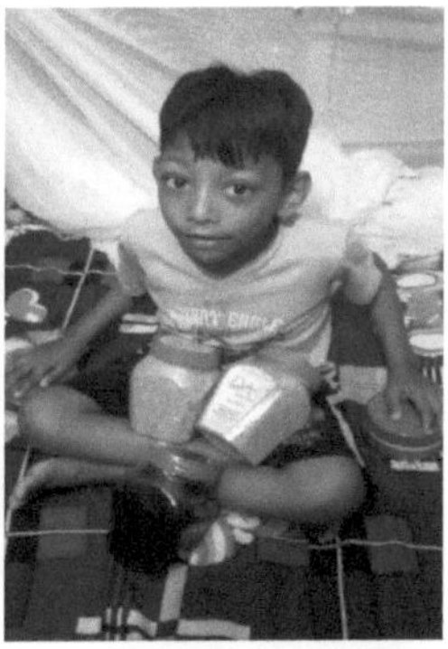
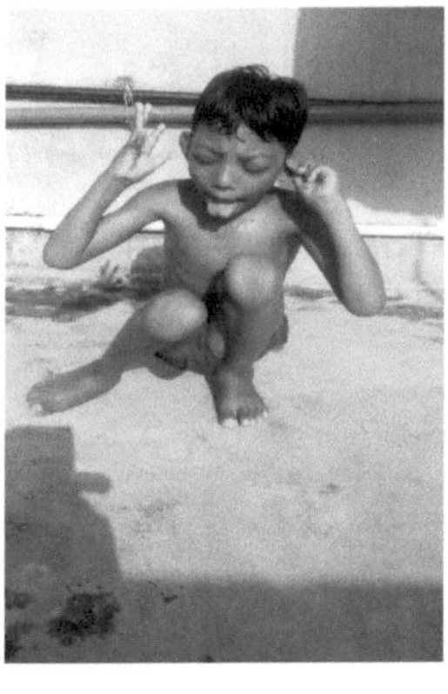
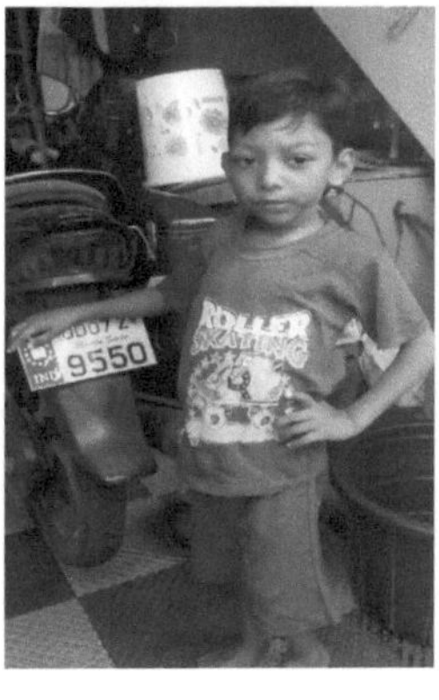

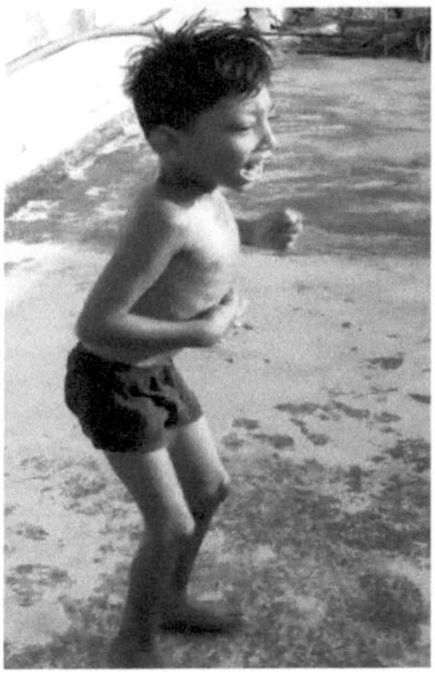

Following were Sandeep Kumar Mohanty parameters before starting Living Water Therapy:

**Frequency of transfusion:** once a month

**Lowest Hemoglobin/ Hb ever recorded:** 4.5

**Medication taken:** Folic Acid, Abrotanum 30 (11ml), Desifer 400

**Physical Symptoms /Discomforts:** weakness, vomitting

They came into our contact on 25-Jul-2022 and started Living Water Therapy.

The present status after starting the therapy

**Frequency of Transfusion:** Nil

**Medications:** Nil

**Physical Symptoms/ Discomforts:** Nil

*Mother and father conveying their thanks to Dr BRC, promise to continue Living Water Therapy as it have given new life to her son. They can see the improvement in his mental health too.*

# 30

Chaitanya Arun Pachangane age 21 yrs, son of Arun (a farmer) and mother Sunanda ( a homemaker), resides in Satara, Maharatsra. Chaitanya Arun Pachangane was diagnosed with thalassemia for the first time at the age of 6 months. Just before the diagnosis he had fever, yellow eyes , weakness. Doctor advised to go for blood test and that was the first time thalassemia was diagnosed. Since then he has been taking treatment at Krishna Hospital,Karad.

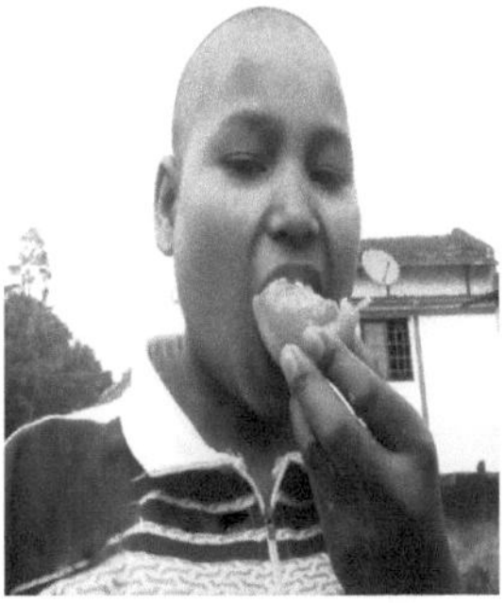
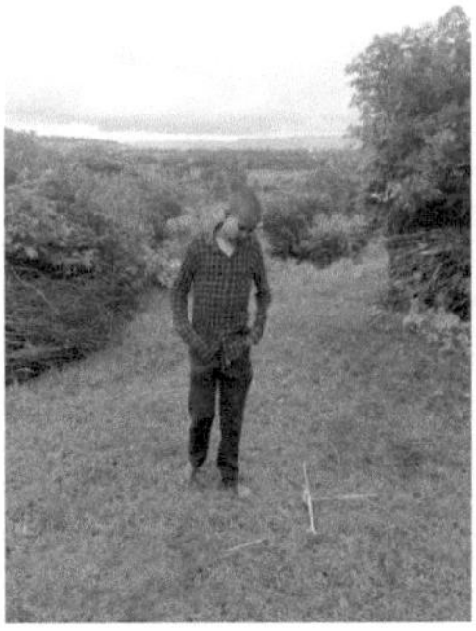
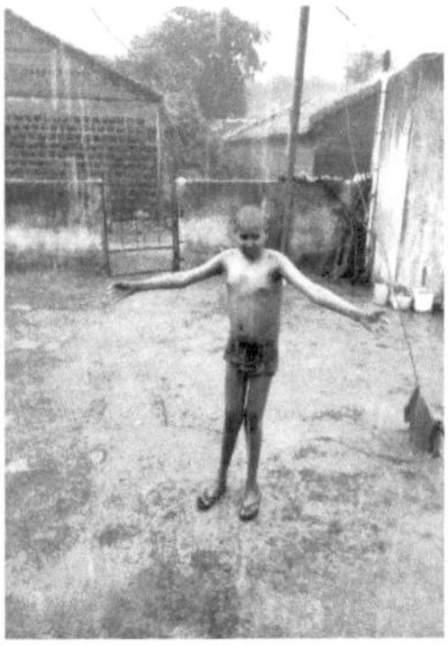

Following were Chaitanya 's parameters before starting Living Water Therapy:

**Frequency of transfusion:** twice a month

**Lowest Hemoglobin/ Hb ever recorded:** 3

Medication taken: deparal,calcium, vitamin c and zinc

**Physical Symptoms /Discomforts:** weakness

They came into our contact on 27-Jul-2022 and started Living Water Therapy.

The present status after starting the therapy

**Frequency of Transfusion:** Nil

**Medications:** Nil

**Physical Symptoms/ Discomforts:** Nil

*Chaitnya shares, "I have read law of attraction. I keep practicing it and I have attracted Dr BRC in my life.Now no disease can touch me without my permission. I no longer consume non-veg food only DIP Diet.*

# 31

Devidas Ukanda Kamble age 25 yrs, son of Ukanda Kamble ( works in fields) and mother Sharda Kamble (a homemaker), resides in Akola, Maharastra. Devidas Ukanda Kamble was diagnosed with thalassemia for the first time at the age of 3 years. Just before the diagnosis he had body pain , fever and weakness, yellow color of the body. Doctor advised to go for blood test and that was the first time thalassemia was diagnosed. Since then he has been taking treatment at Govt Hospital,Akola.

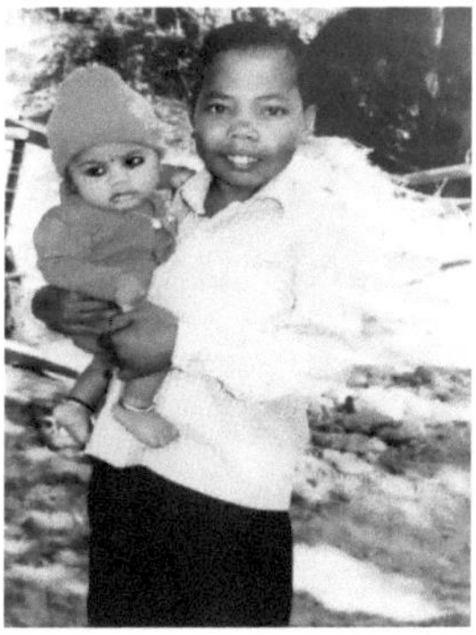

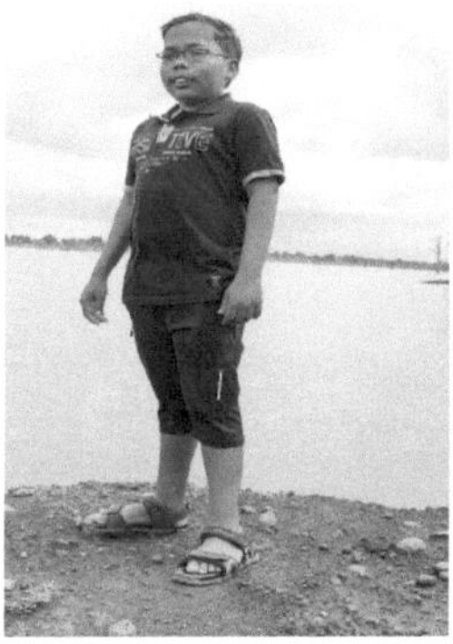

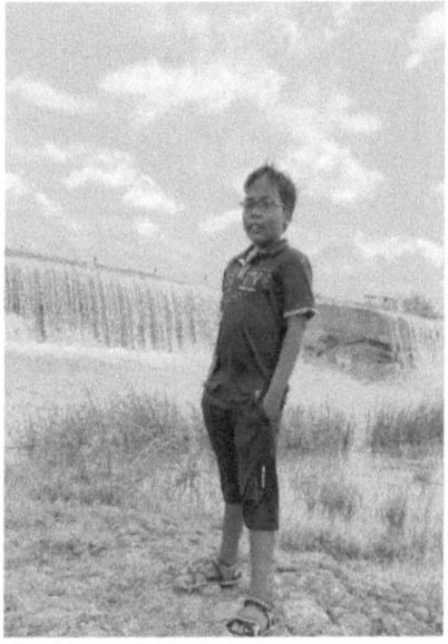

Following were Devidas ‘s parameters before starting Living Water Therapy:

**Frequency of transfusion:** once in 21 days

**Lowest Hemoglobin/ Hb ever recorded:** 3.3

**Medication taken:** folic acid, multi vitamin, cacirol,dezirox, calcium

**Physical Symptoms /Discomforts:** weakness,

They came into our contact on 23-Jul-2022 and started Living Water Therapy.

The present status after starting the therapy

**Frequency of Transfusion:** Nil

**Medications:** Nil

**Physical Symptoms/ Discomforts:** Nil

*Devidas in his chirpy voice conveys many thanks for bringing this joy into his life.*

# 32

Gourav soni age 3.5 yrs, son of Dinesh Soni ( water supply business) and mother Ekta Soni ( a beautician), resides in Faridabaad, Haryana. Gourav soni was diagnosed with thalassemia for the first time at the age of 3.5 months. Just before the diagnosis he had fever, cough & cold and yellowish body. Doctor advised to go for blood test and that was the first time thalassemia was diagnosed. Since then he has been taking treatment at Kalawati, Delhi.

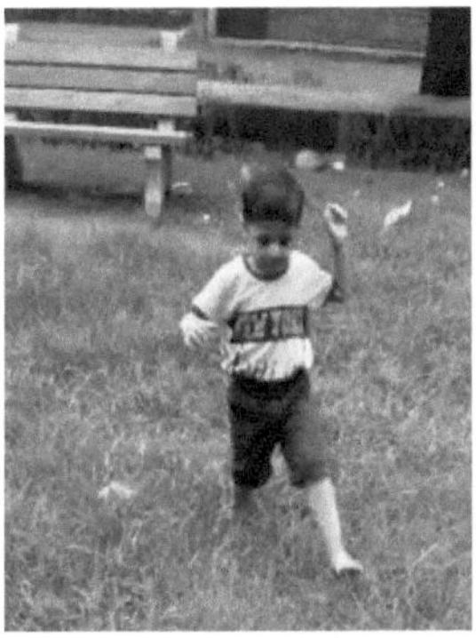
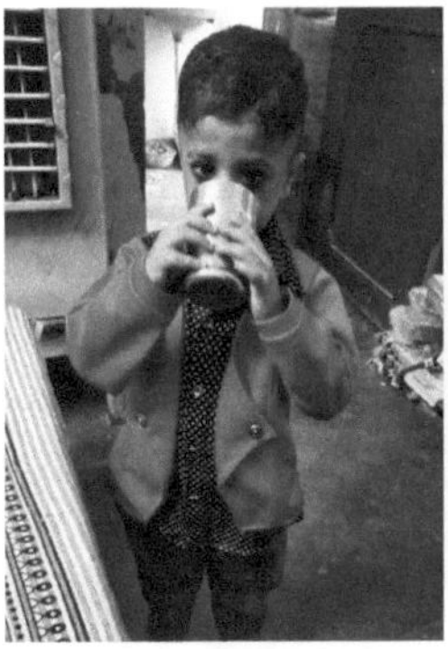
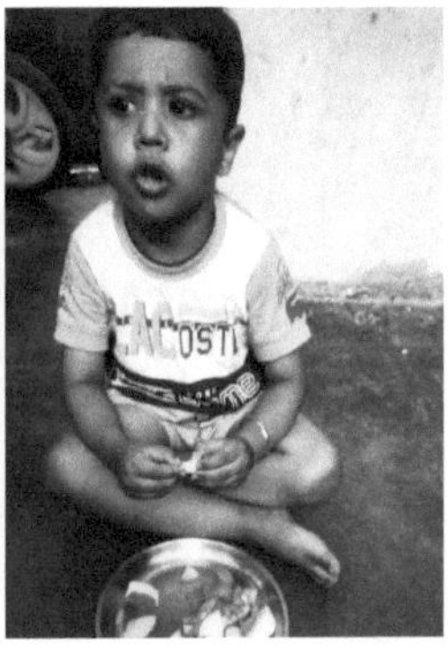

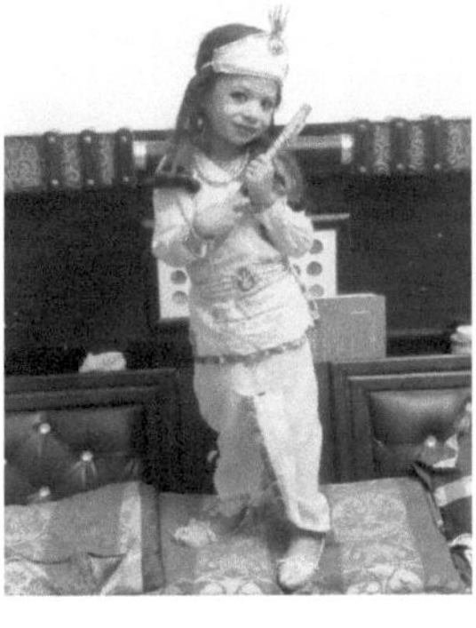
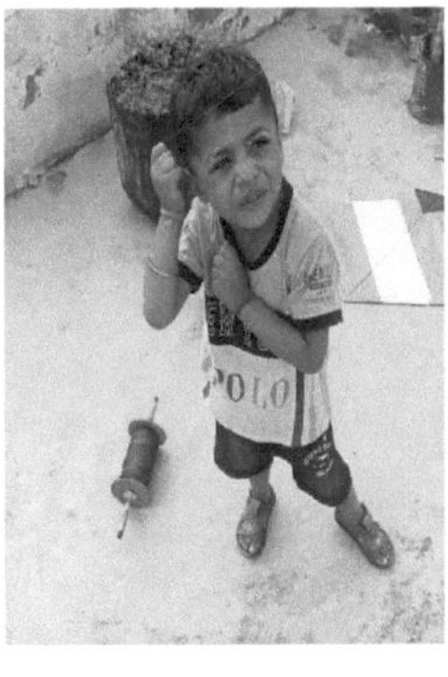
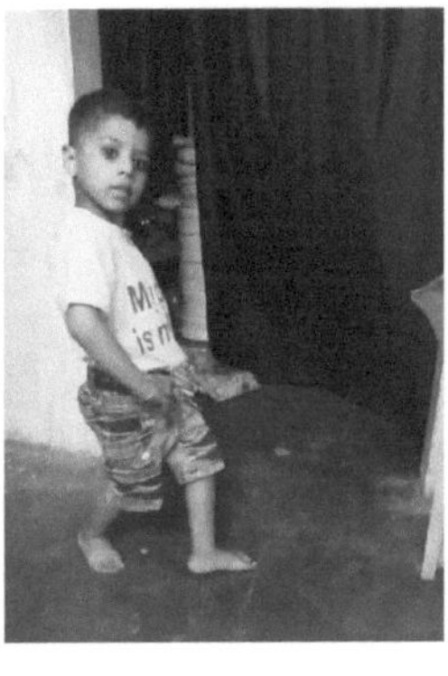

Following were Gourav's parameters before starting Living Water Therapy:

**Frequency of transfusion:** once a month

**Lowest Hemoglobin/ Hb ever recorded:** 6.5

**Medication taken:** folic acid and defirox

Physical Symptoms /Discomforts: weaness and cough

They came into our contact on 26-Jul-2022 and started Living Water Therapy.

The present status after starting the therapy

**Frequency of Transfusion:** Nil

**Medications:** Nil

**Physical Symptoms/ Discomforts:** Nil

*Father shares, "My child is healthy and strong today because of Living Water Therapy. No more blood transfusion. Thank you Dr BRC. & Dr Namita for making this possible.*

# 33

Gungun Goyal age 19 yrs, daughter of Late Mr. Subhash Gupta and mother Lekha Gupta (a teacher in Maharaja Agrasen Public School, Bakhtawarpur), resides in Delhi. Gungun Goyal was diagnosed with thalassemia for the first time at the age of 6 months. Just before the diagnosis she had under weight. Doctor advised to go for blood test and that was the first time thalassemia was diagnosed. Since then she has been taking treatment at Holy Family Hospital, Okhla Road Delhi.

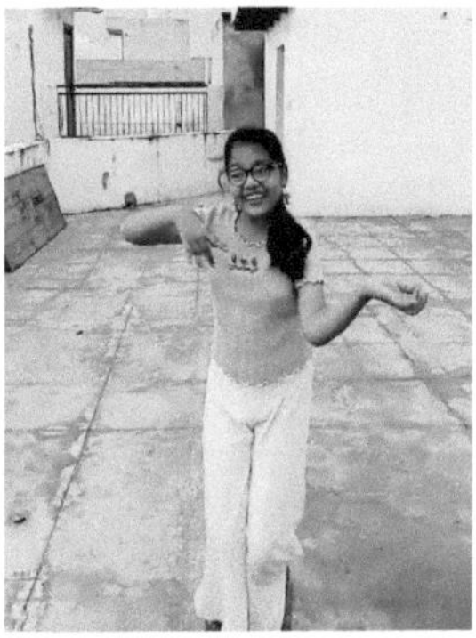
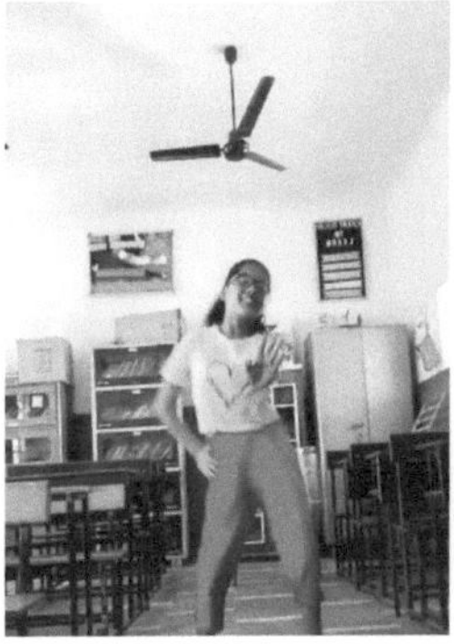
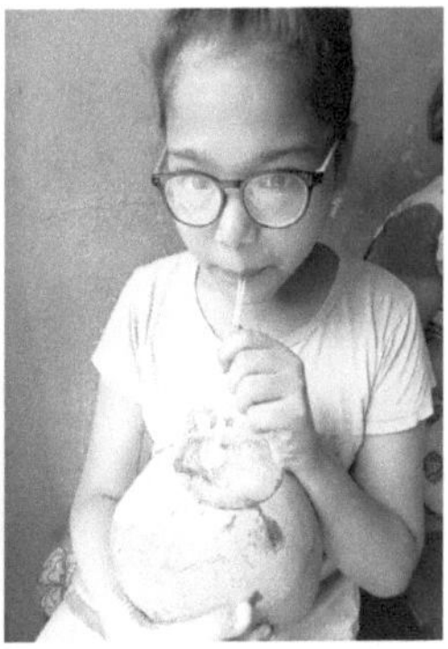

Following were Gungun Goyal parameters before starting Living Water Therapy:

**Frequency of transfusion:** once in 23 days

**Lowest Hemoglobin/ Hb ever recorded:** 3.2

**Medication taken:** calfur,folic acid, shelcal , thyronom , premrine

**Physical Symptoms /Discomforts:** weakness

They came into our contact on 23-Jul-2022 and started Living Water Therapy.

The present status after starting the therapy

**Frequency of Transfusion:** Nil

**Medications:** Nil

**Physical Symptoms/ Discomforts:** Nil

*Gungun shares, "I now feel disease free. Thank you for encouraging me to live meaningful and joyful life."*

# 34

Isha Goyal age 20 yrs, daughter of Late Mr. Subhash Gupta and mother Lekha Gupta ( a teacher in Maharaja Agrasen Public School, Bakhtawarpur), resides in Delhi, . Isha Goyal was diagnosed with thalassemia for the first time at the age of 1 year 7 months. Just before the diagnosis she had fever and swelling on face. Doctor advised to go for blood test and that was the first time thalassemia was diagnosed. Since then she has been taking treatment at Holy Family Hospital, Okhla Road Delhi.

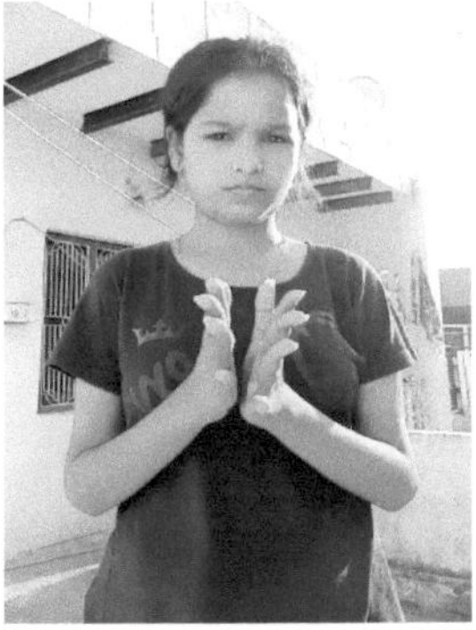

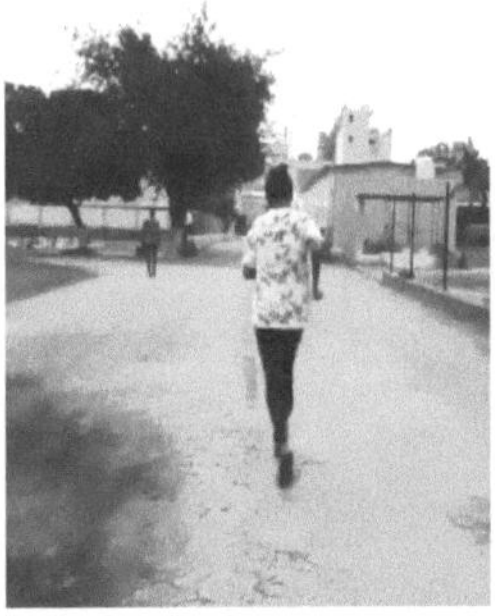

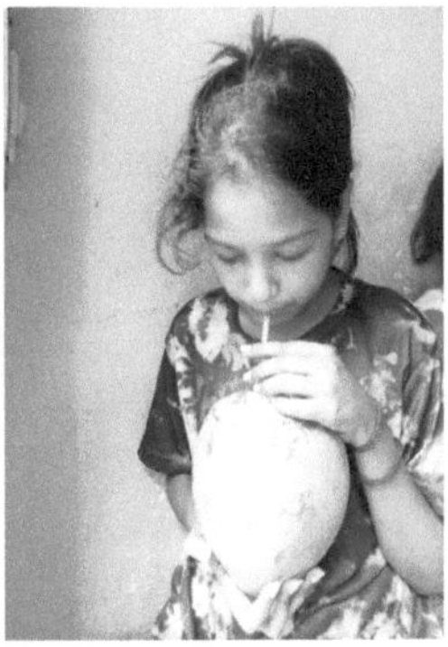

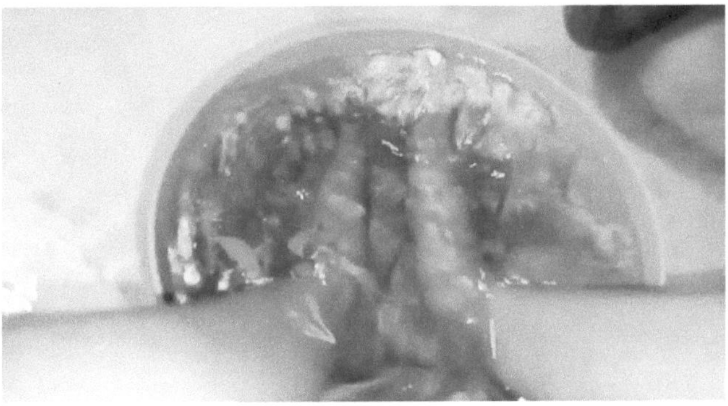

Following were Isha Goyal parameters before starting Living Water Therapy:

**Frequency of transfusion:** once in 23 days

**Lowest Hemoglobin/ Hb ever recorded:** 3.3

**Medication taken:** calfur,folic acid, shelcal, defri Z

**Physical Symptoms /Discomforts:** Nil

They came into our contact on 23-Jul-2022 and started Living Water Therapy.

The present status after starting the therapy

**Frequency of Transfusion:** Nil

**Medications:** Nil

**Physical Symptoms/ Discomforts:** Nil

*Isha comments, " I now feel like a medicine free human!"*

# 35

Ishmeet singh age 9 yrs, son of Gagan (a teacher in an ITI institute) and mother Chanpreet Singh (a homemaker), resides in Delhi, . Ishmeet singh was diagnosed with thalassemia for the first time at the age of 1 year 2 months. Just before the diagnosis he had swelling in stomach, fever , pale yellow skin. Doctor advised to go for blood test and that was the first time thalassemia was diagnosed. Since then he has been taking treatment at Genesis Hospital, Delhi.

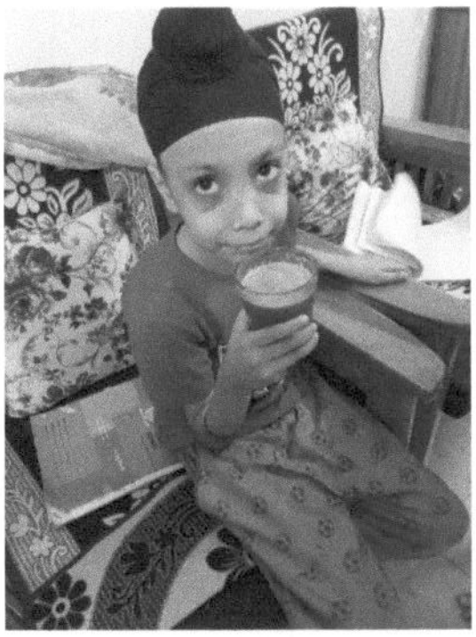
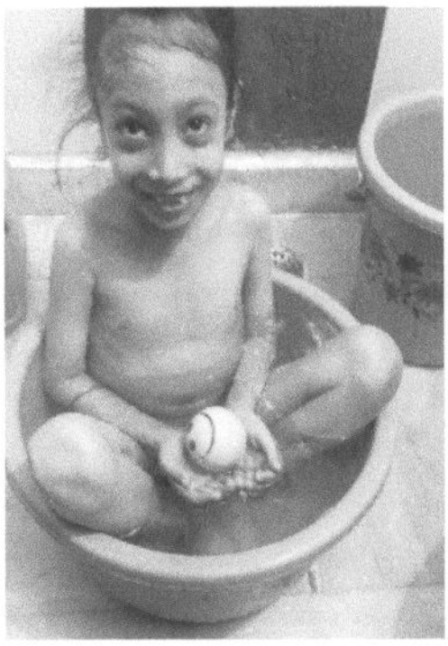
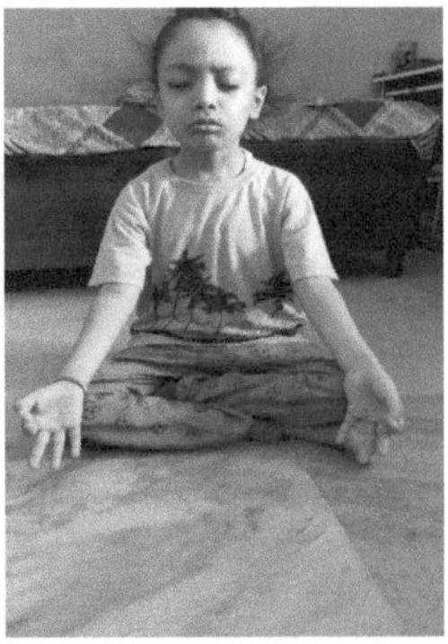
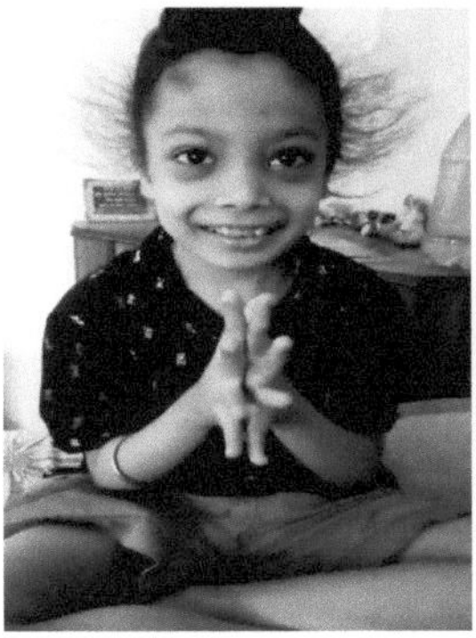
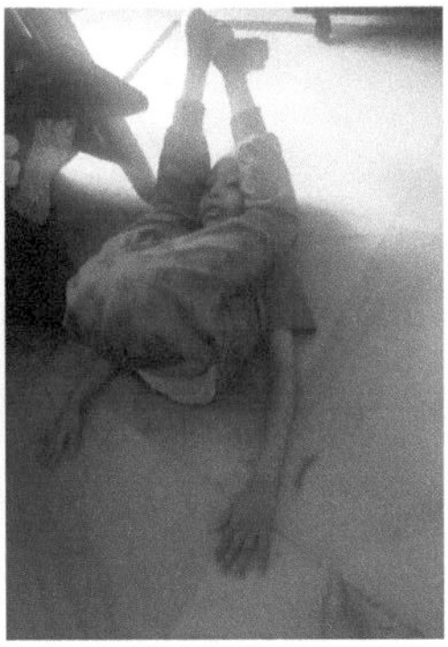
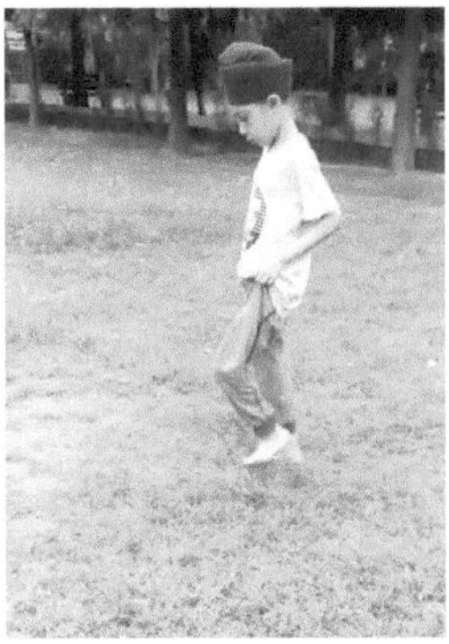

Following were Ishmeet singh parameters before starting Living Water Therapy:

**Frequency of transfusion:** once in 6-8 months

**Lowest Hemoglobin/ Hb ever recorded:** 4.5

Medication taken: hydroxi urea, folic acid, thalix, calcium

Physical Symptoms /Discomforts: pale , fever , infectio, stomach increse with splin

They came into our contact on 31-Jul-2022 and started Living Water Therapy.

The present status after starting the therapy

**Frequency of Transfusion:** Nil

**Medications:** Nil

**Physical Symptoms/ Discomforts:** Nil

*Ishmeet conveys thanks for sharing the knowledge regarding the treatment of thalassemia through Living Water Therapy. He is hopeful about getting rid of this disease permanently.*

# 36

Vedant Pradeep Bansode age 16 years, son of Pradeep (bus conductor) and mother Seema (a homemaker), resides in Osmanabaad, Maharastra. Vedant pradeep Bansode was diagnosed with thalassemia for the first time at the age of 4 months. Just before the diagnosis his body turned white , had loose motion & fever. Doctor advised to go for blood test and that was the first time thalassemia was diagnosed. Since then he has been taking treatment at Unique Hospital , Pune.

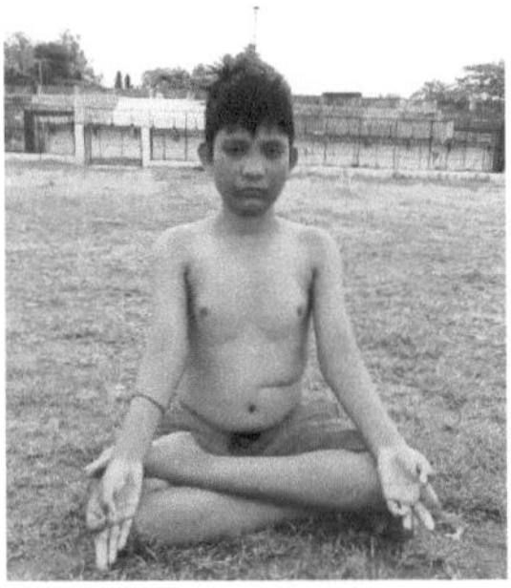
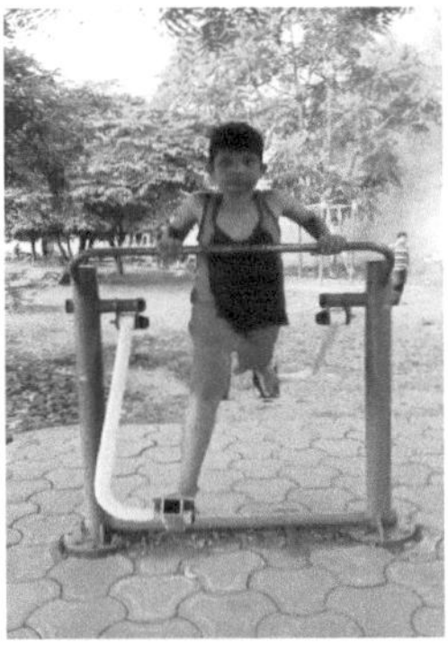
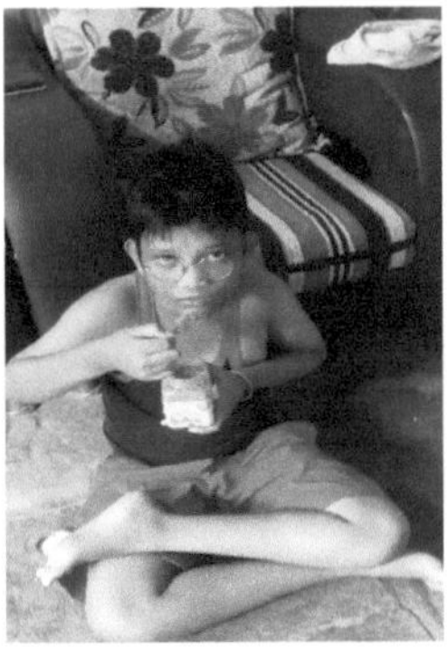
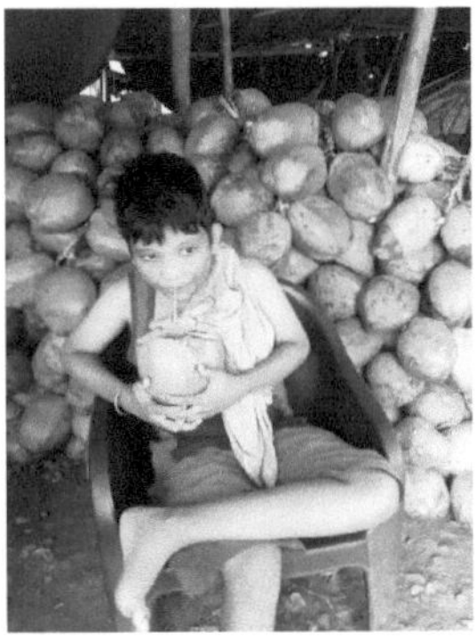
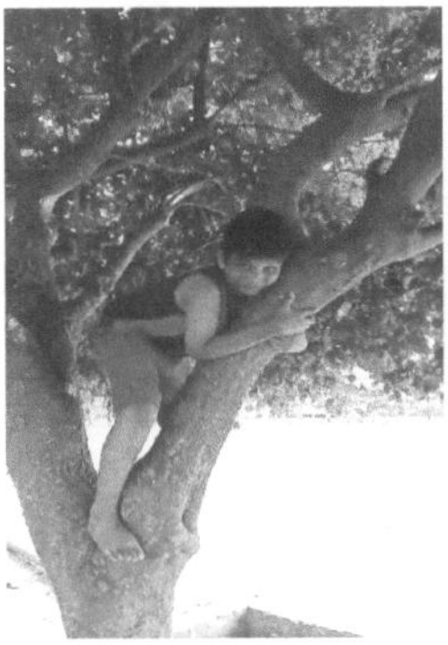
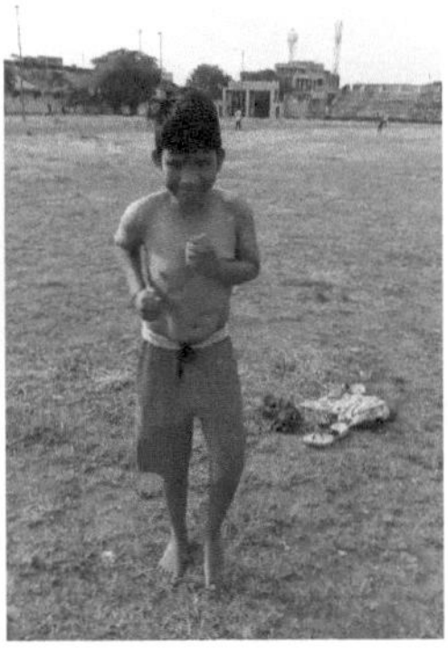

Following were Vedant pradeep Bansode parameters before starting Living Water Therapy:

**Frequency of transfusion:** once in a month

**Lowest Hemoglobin/ Hb ever recorded:** 4.9

**Medication taken:** desiferol,

**Physical Symptoms /Discomforts:** weakness , no hunger

They came into our contact on 28- Jul-2022 and started Living Water Therapy.

The present status after starting the therapy

**Frequency of Transfusion:** Nil

**Medications:** Nil

**Physical Symptoms/ Discomforts:** Nil

# 37

Brajesh Shaw age 2.5 years, son of Sabhya Sachi ( business- tent house) and mother Shivli Shah(a homemaker), resides in Jamsedpur, Jharkhand. Brajesh Shaw was diagnosed with thalassemia for the first time at the age of 7 months. Just before the diagnosis he had fever. Doctor advised to go for blood test and that was the first time thalassemia was diagnosed. Since then he has been taking treatment at Baropada Hospital, Odisha.

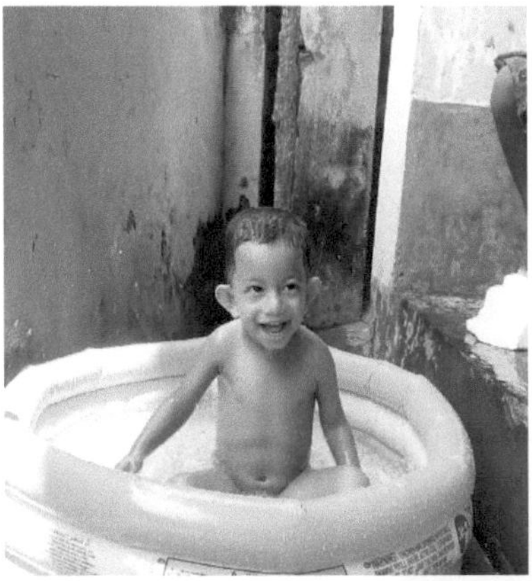

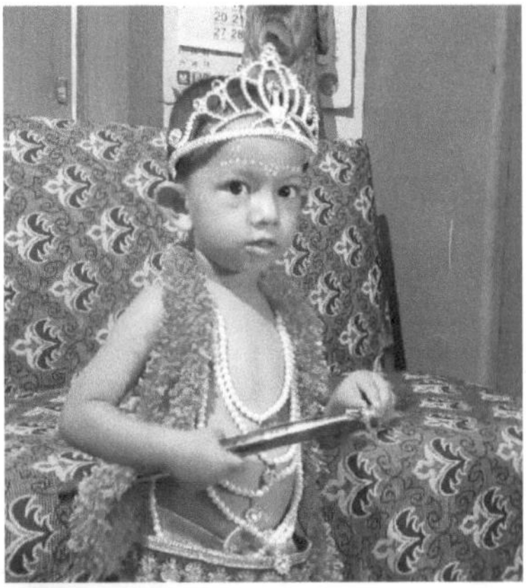

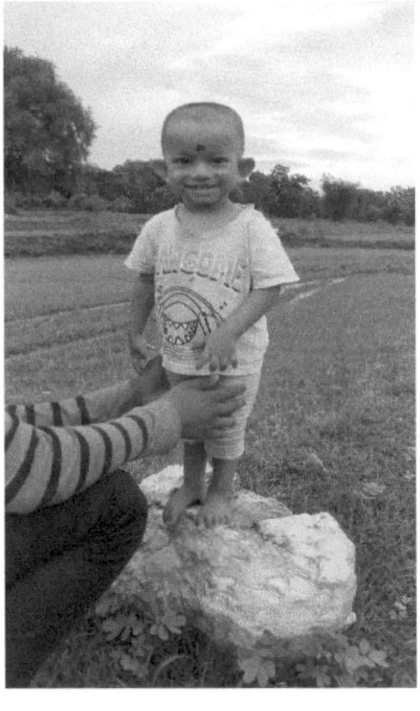

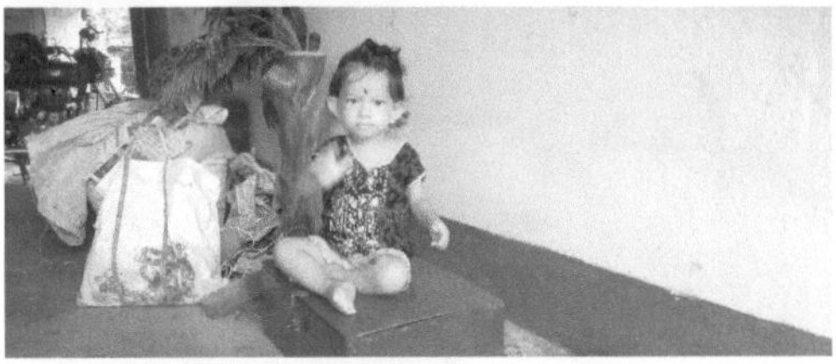

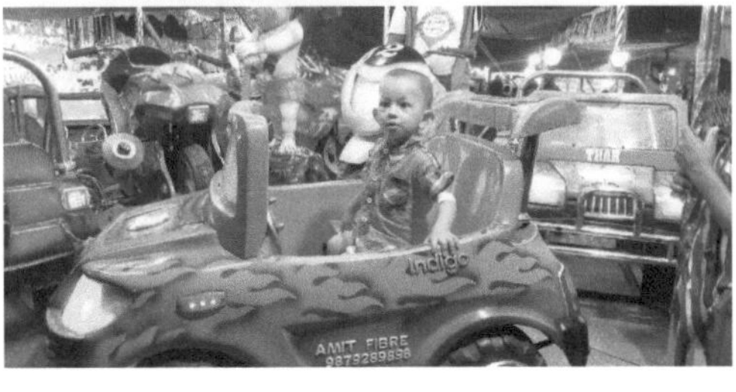

Following were Brajesh Shaw parameters before starting Living Water Therapy:

**Frequency of transfusion:** once in a month

**Lowest Hemoglobin/ Hb ever recorded:** 4.6

**Medication taken:** folic acid

Physical Symptoms /Discomforts: weakness, ferver, no hunger

They came into our contact on 9-Aug-2022 and started Living Water Therapy.

The present status after starting the therapy

**Frequency of Transfusion:** Nil

**Medications:** Nil

**Physical Symptoms/ Discomforts:** Nil

*Father shares, "A ray of hope is visible through Living Water Therapy. Every month we were taking the child for blood transfusion but now it's beyond 1 month and child is healthy with no signs of any requirement for blood transfusion."*

# 38

Pankaj Sardana age 34 years, son of Inderjit Sardana (driver) and mother Priya Sardana (runs a beauty parlour at home), resides in Mohali, Punjab. Pankaj Sardana was diagnosed with thalassemia for the first time at the age of 1.5 years. Just before the diagnosis he had loose motion and weakness. Doctor advised to go for blood test and that was the first time thalassemia was diagnosed. Since then he has been taking treatment in a hospital in Karnal .

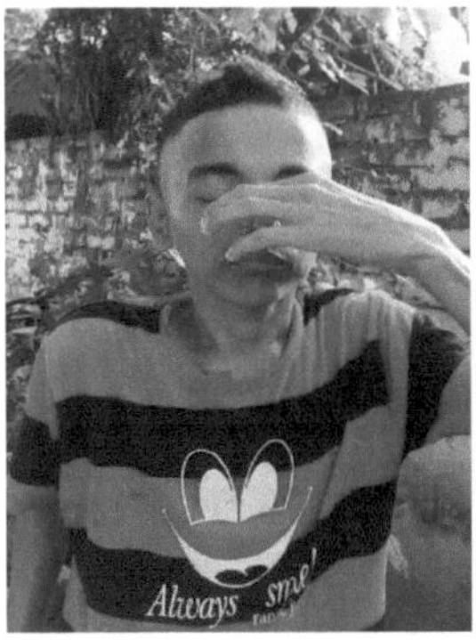

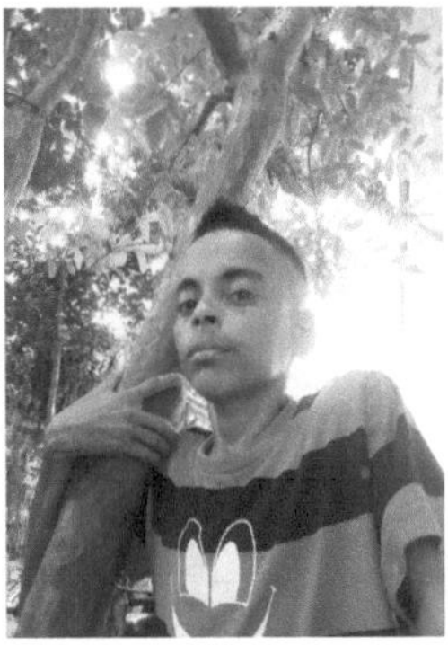
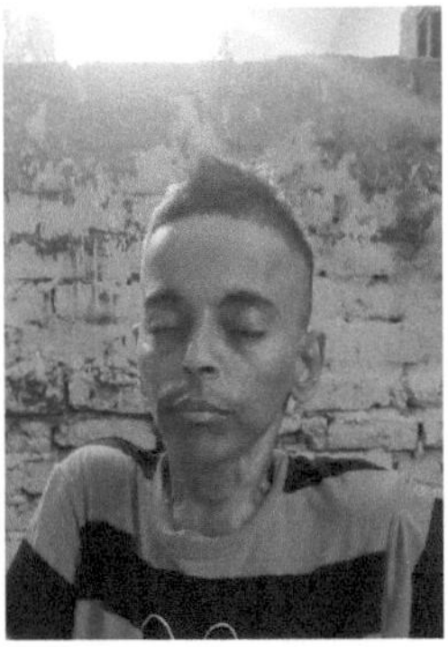

Following were Pankaj Sardana parameters before starting Living Water Therapy:

**Frequency of transfusion:** Once in 15 days

**Lowest Hemoglobin/ Hb ever recorded:** 6

**Medication taken:** desirox, folic acid , calfur

**Physical Symptoms /Discomforts:** Nil

They came into our contact on 26-Jul-2022 and started Living Water Therapy.

The present status after starting the therapy

**Frequency of Transfusion:** Nil

**Medications:** Nil

**Physical Symptoms/ Discomforts:** Nil

# 39

Siddharth Bharti age 8 yrs, son of Vikram Kesri Bharti (private job) and mother Swagatika Bharti (a teacher ), resides in, Cuttak, Odisha . Siddharth Bharti was diagnosed with thalassemia for the first time at the age of 6 months. Just before the diagnosis parents observed his pale and whitish body color . Doctor advised to go for blood test and that was the first time thalassemia was diagnosed. Since then he has been taking treatment at Apollo- Buwaneshwar.

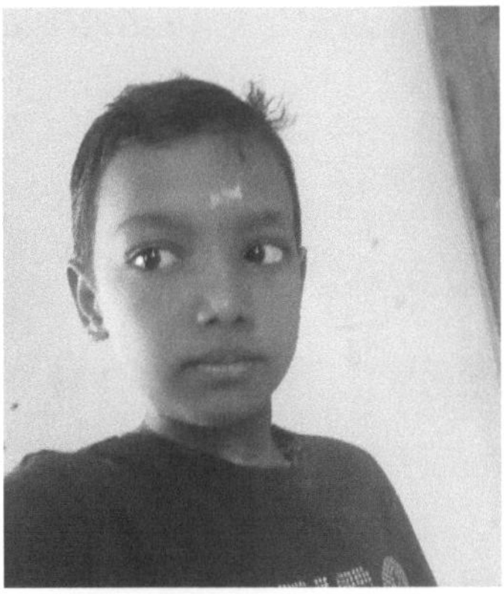

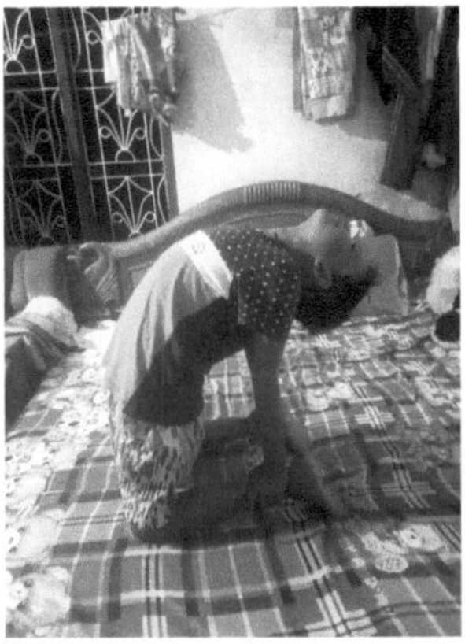

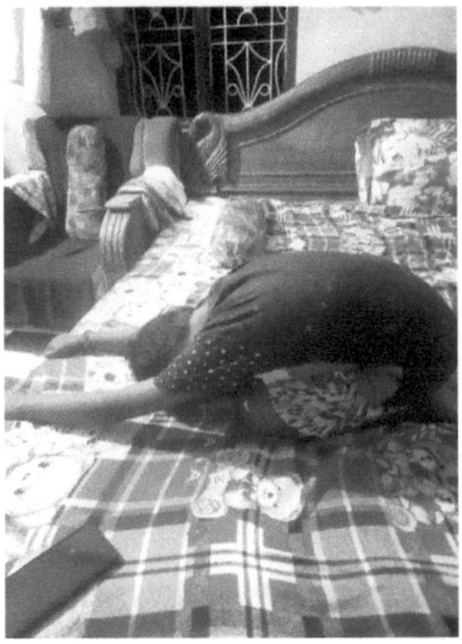

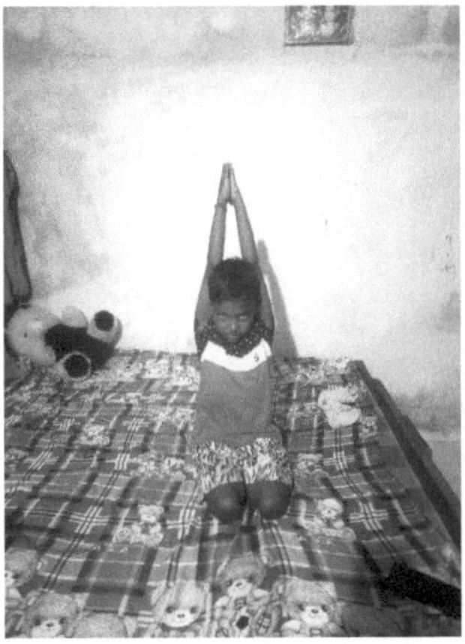

Following were Siddharth Bharti parameters before starting Living Water Therapy:

**Frequency of transfusion:** once in 15 days

**Lowest Hemoglobin/ Hb ever recorded:** 5.5

**Medication taken:** defrijet, multivitamin, zincovit, folic acid

**Physical Symptoms /Discomforts:** pale body

They came into our contact on 17-Aug-2022 and started Living Water Therapy.

The present status after starting the therapy

**Frequency of Transfusion:** Nil

**Medications:** difrijet

**Physical Symptoms/ Discomforts:** Nil

# 40

Farhan Akhtar age 11 years, son of Md Akhtar Hussain ( runs his own business) and mother Tarannum Perween ( a teacher), resides in Bokaro, Jharkhand. Farhan Akhtar was diagnosed with thalassemia for the first time at the age of 1 year. Just before the diagnosis he had consistent high fever. Doctor advised me to go for a blood test and that was the first time thalassemia was diagnosed. Since then he has been taking treatment at BGH Bokaro.

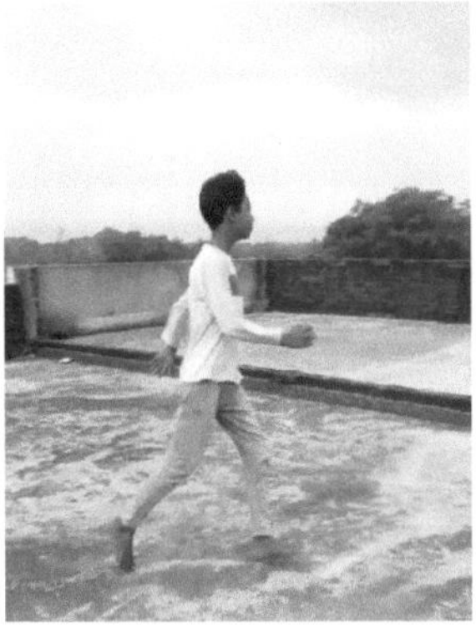

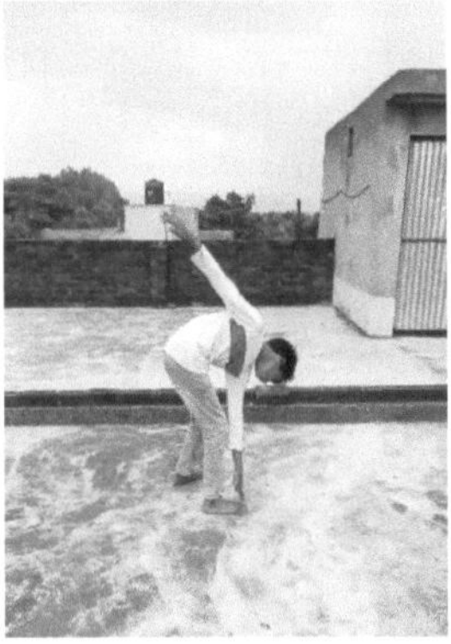

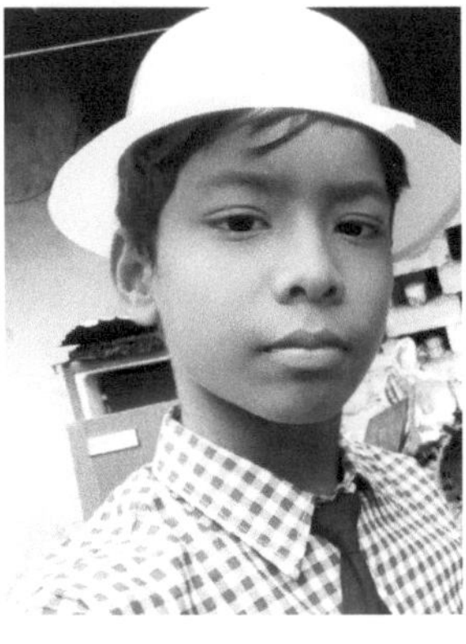

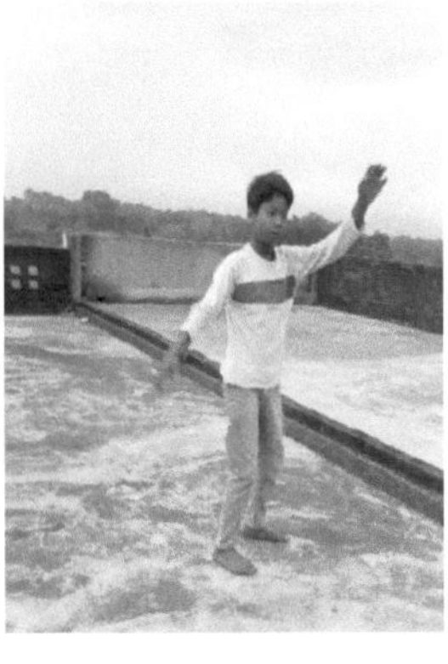

Following were Farhan Akhtar parameters before starting Living Water Therapy:

**Frequency of transfusion:** once every three months

**Lowest Hemoglobin/ Hb ever recorded:** 3

**Medication taken:** Liv-52, Aciloc rd, Folvit, Ostocalcium, Cell activator, Evion 400, Hydrea 500, Menabol,

**Physical Symptoms /Discomforts:** Nil

They came into our contact on 11-Aug-2022 and started Living Water Therapy.

The present status after starting the therapy

**Frequency of Transfusion:** Nil

**Medications:** Nil

**Physical Symptoms/ Discomforts:** Nil

*Mother shares, "Vellore hospital straightaway asked for bone marrow transplant and declared no other way if we wanted to keep the child alive. We had lost all hope. We then took treatment from Kolkata and started medications. Farhan needed transfusion only once a year with this treatment and continued medicines. This year he needed 3-4 transfusion in the beginning. Then we came Across Living Water Therapy program. Since then we are hopeful that Farhan will be completely healed. We can see the difference in the child. The child is following DIP diet happily."*

# From the 1st Page of 1st Chapter

I met Ravi Valecha for the first time in my Faridabad office.

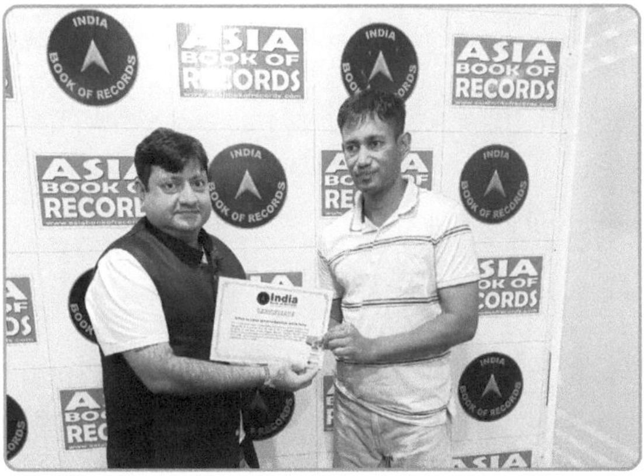


He has a very pleasing and jovial personality. As told by him while growing up, he established himself in films and was known as Master Ravi for quite some time until he established himself as Ravi Valecha soon enough. He also worked in many TV shows which became quite popular. After acting in a string of films, he decided to make a career in hospitality and pursued Masters in Hospitality and International Business from National Institute of Management, Ahmedabad. He now offers his hospitality services to India's top private sector banks. He also gives training on personality development and other skills to children who aspire to make it big in hospitality.

# Books by Dr. Biswaroop Roy Chowdhury

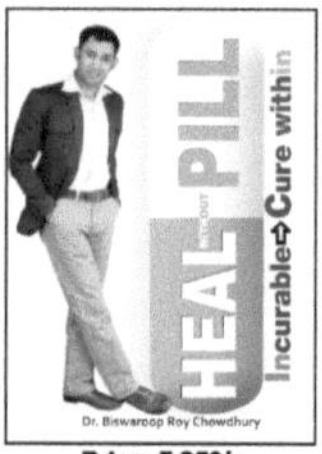


**Price: ₹ 250/-**
(Courier charges extra)

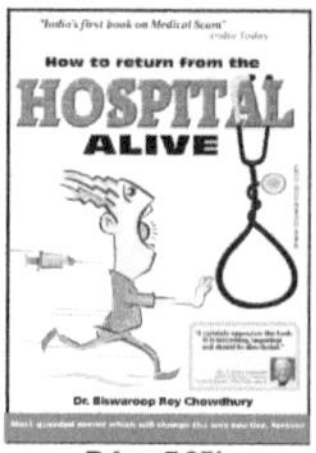


**Price: ₹ 95/-**
(Courier charges extra)

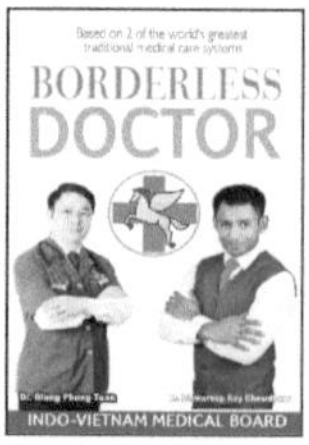


**Price: ₹ 150/-**
(Courier charges extra)

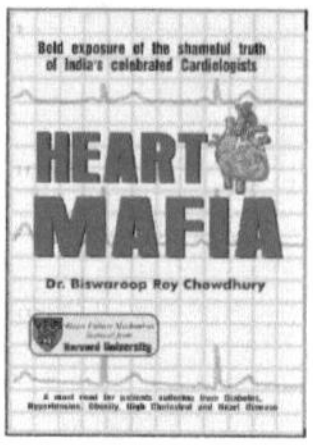


**Price: ₹ 150/-**
(Courier charges extra)

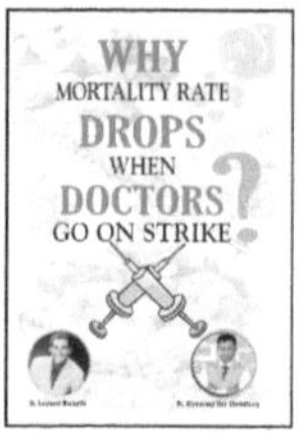


**Price: ₹200/-**
(Courier charges extra)

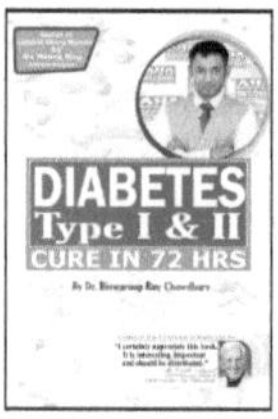


**Price: ₹150/-**
(Courier charges extra)

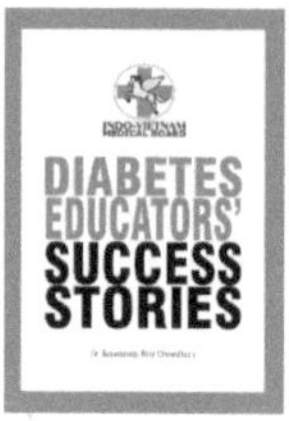


**Price: ₹ 195/-**
(Courier charges extra)

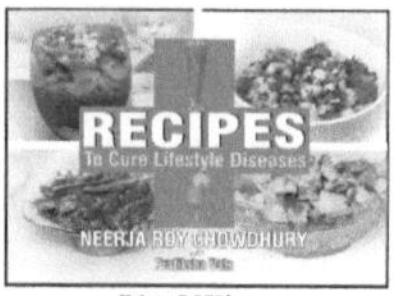


**Price: ₹ 350/-**
(Courier charges extra)

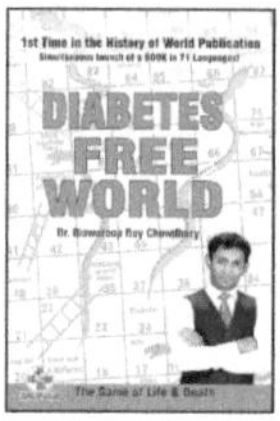


**Price: ₹ 100/-**
(Courier charges extra)

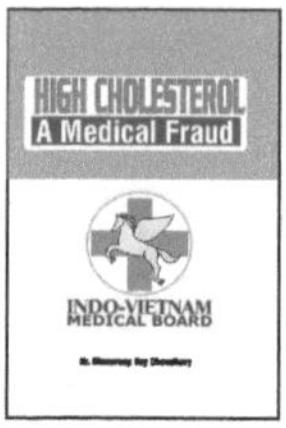


**Price: ₹ 100/-**
(Courier charges extra)

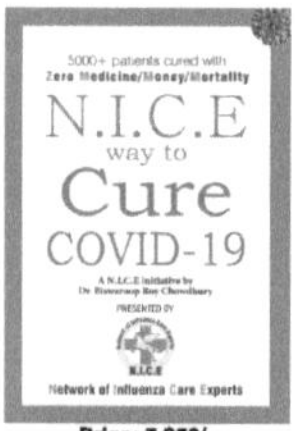


**Price: ₹ 250/-**
(Courier charges extra)

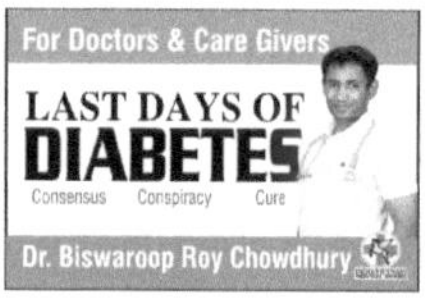


**Price: ₹ 150/-**
(Courier charges extra)

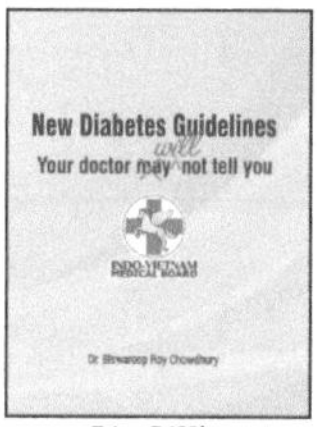


**Price: ₹ 100/-**
(Courier charges extra)

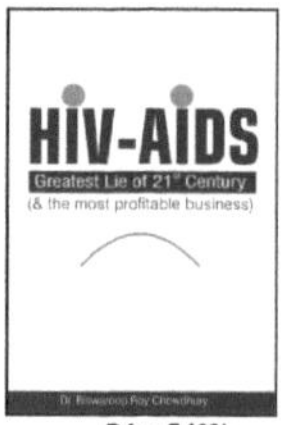


**Price: ₹ 100/-**
(Courier charges extra)

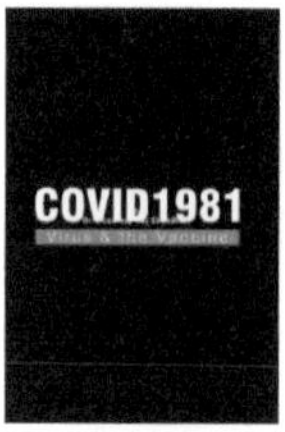


**Price: ₹ 175/-**
(Courier charges extra)

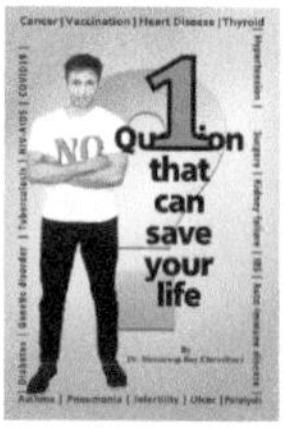


**Price: ₹ 175/-**
(Courier charges extra)

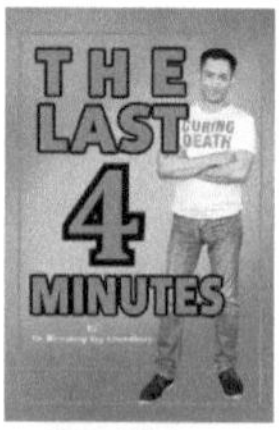


**Price: ₹ 150/-**
(Courier charges extra)

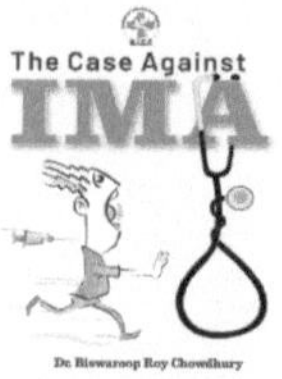


**Price: ₹ 150/-**
(Courier charges extra)

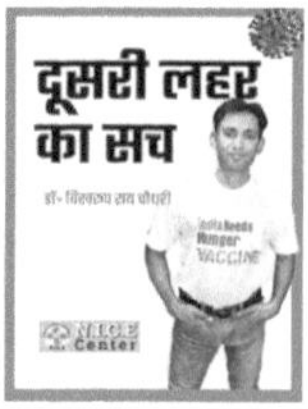


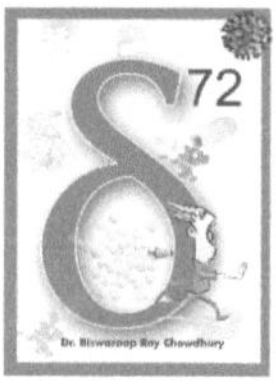


**Price: ₹150/-**
(Courier charges extra)

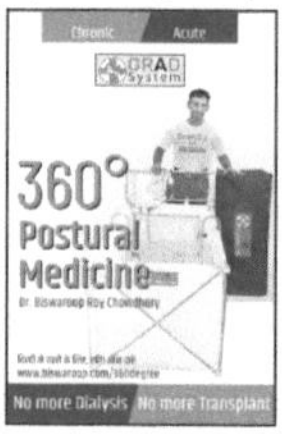


**Price: ₹ 225/-**
(Courier charges extra)

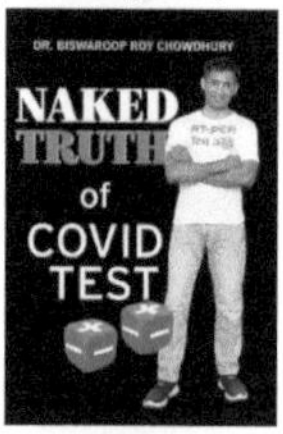


**Price: ₹ 200/-**
(Courier charges extra)

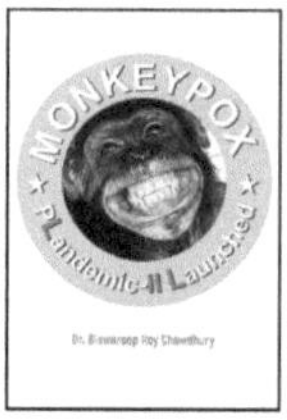


**Price: ₹ 100/-**
(Courier charges extra)

**Buy online at: www.biswaroop.com/shop**

**Dynamic Memory Pvt. Ltd.**

B-121, 2nd Floor, Green Fields, Faridabad-121010 (Haryana), Mob.:+91-9312286540

E-mail:biswaroop@biswaroop.com

**(Available in Hindi/English, in all leading onlinestores)**

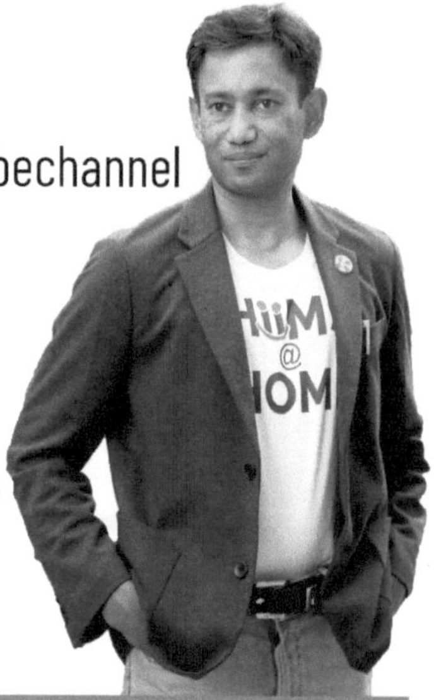

## Let every morning be the Hunza Morning

**If you have decided to pick only one of my suggestions for the sake of your health, then take this suggestion:**

Stop consuming tea specially, morning tea. The early morning tea makes the inner lining of your intestinal wall acidic, as after a long night of fasting your stomach is empty and craving for food. An acidic stomach on a regular basis is the single biggest cause of all kind of inflammatory and lifestyle diseases including arthritis, Diabetes etc.

**How to stop craving of tea ⟶ Switch to Hunza Tea**

Hunza Civilization: Hunza people are the Indians living at extreme northwest of India in Hindu Kush range. They are known to be one of the world's healthiest civilizations, often living up to the age of 110 years.

### How to prepare Hunza Tea (serves four):

**Ingredients:**

- 12 Mint leaves(Pudina)
- 8 Basil Leaves(Tulsi)
- 4 Green cardamom (Elaichi)
- 2 gm Cinnamon (Dalchini)
- 20 gm Ginger (Adrak)
- 20 gm Jaggery (Gur)

**Instructions:**

- Take 4 cups of water in a tea pan
- Add all ingredients, simmer it for 10mins
- Add a dash of lemon juice and serve hot or cold

**For those who are too lazy to collect the above ingredients (to make their own hunza tea) may order**

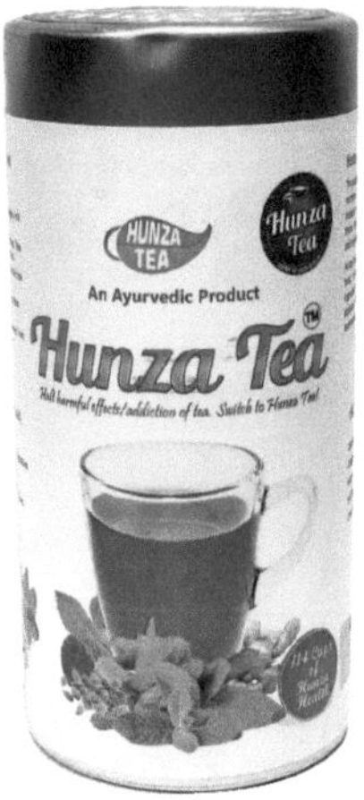


*114 Cups of Hunza Health*

₹ 400/-
(Including Courier charges)

**You may place your order at:**

**Dynamic Memory Pvt. Ltd.**
**B-121, 2nd Floor, Green Fields,**
**Faridabad (Haryana)**
**Mobile No.:+91-9312286540,**
**E-mail: biswaroop@biswaroop.com**

**Log on to www.biswaroop.com/shop to buy products**

Printed in the USA
CPSIA information can be obtained
at www.ICGtesting.com
LVHW061553181123
764050LV00090B/40